MORE PRAISE FOR YVONNE K. FULBRIGHT

"Dr. Yvonne is a smart, hip and totally with-it sexuality expert who's been helping people achieve healthy, happy, fulfilling relationships for years. So when she's giving you great new sex advice like this, take it!"

—**Amy Spencer**, author of *Meeting Your Half-Orange: An Utterly Upbeat Guide to Using Dating Optimism to Find Your Perfect Match*

"Yvonne was able to design a fun, sexy, no-nonsense erotic program to help singles and couples explore and embrace sex talk. Yvonne coaches readers in the comprehensive range of A–Z topics that erotic talk entails. Her approach provides the opportunity for readers to navigate their personal situation to ultimately assess if their relationship is a safe environment for exploration."

—**Amy Levine, M.A.**, sex coach, certified sexuality educator, and founder of sexedsolutions.com

Text © 2010 Yvonne K. Fulbright

First published in the USA in 2010 by
Quiver, a member of
Quayside Publishing Group
100 Cummings Center
Suite 406-L
Beverly, MA 01915-6101
www.quiverbooks.com

14 13 12 11 10   1 2 3 4 5

ISBN-13: 978-1-59233-387-5
ISBN-10: 1-59233-387-7

Library of Congress Cataloging-in-Publication Data
Fulbright, Yvonne K.
  Sultry sex talk to seduce any lover : lust-inducing lingo and
titillating tactics for maximizing your pleasure / Yvonne K.
Fulbright.
    p. cm.
  ISBN-13: 978-1-59233-387-5
  ISBN-10: 1-59233-387-7
  1. Sex. 2. Sex instruction. 3. Interpersonal communication. 4.
Intimacy (Psychology) 5. Verbal behavior. 6. Erotica. I. Title.
  HQ23.F85 2009
  613.9'6--dc22
                                    2009040596

Cover design by Landers Miller Design
Book design by Holtz Design

Printed and bound in Singapore

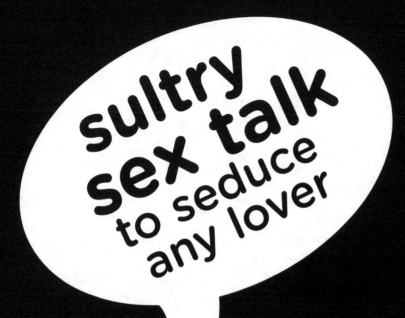

sultry sex talk
to seduce any lover

LUST-INDUCING LINGO
AND TITILLATING TACTICS FOR
MAXIMIZING YOUR PLEASURE

Yvonne K. Fulbright, Ph.D.

QUIVER

For Bianca, Marci, and Tiffany. For always letting me "talk your ears off" about love, sex, and relationships.

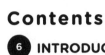

Contents

INTRODUCTION
Erotic Talk:
Orgasm-Inducing
Lip Service

"I wish you were snuggling up against me right now. I'd love to be caressing your hot bod, slowly making love to every inch of you, driving you soooo crazy with my rock hard cock."

"Be good and sit still. I'm in charge now."

"You are the air I breathe."

"Do you like that? I promised you wouldn't be disappointed."

"I just got off thinking about how your warm, wet pussy spasmed around me last weekend."

"I can't get enough of you."

"Play with me."

"You're such a naughty tease. Now it's your turn to shudder with sensations. Straddle my face so I can feast on you."

"I've been meaning to tell you . . . I love you."

"Don't stop kissing me."

"Tell me that fantasy again."

When it comes to

revving up sexual desire or transforming one's sex life, few give enough kudos to the other kind of "aural." Involving much more than "dirty talk," erotic talk offers new ways to intensify and redefine your sexual intimacy, helping you and your lover maintain, crank up, and recharge passion for years to come. Whether in or out of the bedroom, turning up the vamp volume can set the mood, heighten desire, strengthen bonds, and take sex to a whole new level of excitement and exploration.

INTRODUCING EROTIC TALK into your relationship has the power to:

➜ Stimulate more than your imaginations for greater enthrallment and sexual satisfaction
➜ Intensify sensations and the overall sexual experience
➜ Heighten your orgasms, taking you to places previously unknown
➜ Boost your level of intimacy, sharing, and connection
➜ Add creativity, novelty, and inspiration

Tongue action truly does take on a whole new meaning in *Sultry Sex Talk to Seduce Any Lover: Lust-Inducing Lingo and Titillating Tactics for Maximizing Your Pleasure.* Offering both couples and singles a one-of-a-kind approach to sexual communication, this book is packed with flirtalicious exercises, vital information, situations that beg for erotic talk, and sexy sound bites that will bring the art of talking sexy to your sex life. This work promises to:

➜ Supercharge your sex life, making it hotter, more satisfying, and more intense via skillful erotic talk in various situations, including sexy role-playing
➜ Rev up your lust life with luscious tongue-lashings as we explore the different types of erotic talk at your disposal for flirting, foreplay, main play, and afterplay
➜ Provide you with effective erotic communication strategies for increasing your sexual repertoire and leaving a lasting impression
➜ Equip you with the vocabulary, inspiration, and practices needed to eliminate bedroom boredom and deliver erotic talk with confidence anytime, anywhere
➜ Empower you to initiate more sex and the kind of sex you want, helping you to overcome any discomfort, intimidation, or embarrassment in communicating about your needs, revealing your fantasies and desires, and taking charge in and out of your boudoir

Enhanced by quizzes, checklists, self-evaluations, and feedback from an erotic talk survey,* *Sultry Sex Talk to Seduce Any Lover: Lust-Inducing Lingo and Titillating Tactics for Maximizing Your Pleasure* offers you a fresh, coordinated action plan to achieve your personal goals. No matter what your gender or sexual orientation, get ready for a sex-positive sex communication crash course in easy aural execution. The passion plan goes as follows:

Chapter 1: Getting Ready for Erotic Talk

This first chapter looks at what's required of a sexual relationship, casual or serious, when it comes to practicing erotic talk. Using a checklist, you will be asked to size up essentials for launching such sex play (e.g., good general communication and a solid trust component). The Erotic Talk Preferences Quiz helps you figure out your potential for pleasuring. We lay the foundation for erotic talk and making you sexually satisfied by establishing ground rules. The dos and don'ts of talking sexy are discussed, including the need for boundaries and deciding what's dirty versus degrading and a turn-on versus a turn-off.

Chapter 2: "Coming" into Your Own with Erotic Talk

Focusing solely on you, chapter 2 tackles issues that can affect your game, such as fear and embarrassment. Learn the art of erotic talk as you explore various sources of inspiration, warming up with exercises to help you reach greater feelings of ease and empowerment.

Chapter 3: Practice Makes Perfect

Chapter 3 cultivates your carnal connection with a run-through of everything you need to practice erotic talk and tackle barriers to erotic discourse and sharing. Exercises and tips for how to communicate about sex (and how not to) are given, with special focus on sexual compatibility

---

* I did not collect the names of the Erotic Talk Survey participants to protect their anonymity. The names that appear in the book have been randomly selected, and any that bear a potential likeness to a real person are purely coincidental.

and letting your tongue take charge. Here, erotic feedback is where it's at, including a scintillating show-and-tell for make-no-mistakes-about-what-I-want erotic talk.

Chapter 4: Firing Up Foreplay
Chapter 4 focuses on the role of erotic talk during foreplay, including the full-force effect of body language. Different sexual scenarios are delved into, as you flirt and play before and after sex.

Chapter 5: Erotic Talk Tech-Style
Chapter 5 looks at the different types of tech-sex, including email, text messaging, instant messaging, cyber-sex, and phone sex. The many hotter-than-hot methods for seducing your partner throughout the day are discussed in building anticipation.

Chapter 6: Sexplorations: Where Will Your Tongue Take You?
Chapter 6 dives into fantasy and role-playing made more thrilling when erotic talk is added to the mix. From sharing your wildest fantasies to practicing bondage and S&M, this chapter encourages readers to push their erotic envelope and stoke their sexual imaginations.

Chapter 7: Tackling Issues That Can Trump Your Game
Chapter 7 helps you nip issues in the bud for good by examining personal inhibitors and relationship issues that hinder sexual expression. Here, you get a handle on these intimacy intruders so that you can talk your way to bliss in the bedroom and beyond.

Meet Your Erotic Talk Coach

I was immediately intrigued by this book project, especially since I'm quite familiar with the books out there about spicing things up with sex communication. Because these works largely focus on issues like how to communicate about low desire or ask about your partner's needs, I wanted to focus on an equally important but often lacking factor in the mouth moves department: lust-inducing lingo. And what a titillating task it proved to be. Let's just say that researching erotic literature isn't your average day on the job, even when you're a sex expert: One can have trouble staying on task . . .

This project has been a thrill in that it is the perfect opportunity to educate readers about the sex communication issues I see daily as a sex educator. Over the years, in writing sex columns and blogs, working with the media as a sexologist resource, teaching or guest lecturing at universities, and answering emails posted to websites like mine (www.sensualfusion.com and www. sexualitysource.com), I've fielded a

plethora of questions and concerns. And there's a common theme that underlies all of these most intimate inquiries and issues: the need for lovers to learn how to communicate effectively—and erotically—with each other.

As a result, much of the content, recommendations, and assignments in this book are drawn from my professional observations and experiences as a sexologist and sex educator with academic degrees in human sexuality, health education, psychology, and sociology, with specializations in sex communication and sexual and reproductive health. Some of it's just too hot not to handle, from my point of view.

Both personally and professionally, I'm all about fostering a holistic, whole-person, sensually fused approach to better sex, stronger relationships, and overall life improvement. So like a good fitness trainer, I'm here to keep you focused, challenged, and motivated in improving your performance, enhancing your sex life, and reaching your erotic talk and personal development goals. I'm here to refute unhealthy social messaging about erotic talk, reframe negative messages about talking sexy, and give you permission to pursue what's right for you by creating more awareness and empowering you.

But ultimately, your satisfaction and learning will come from within as you do your own work. The learning and action required to fulfill your sexy talk desires and intentions are all up to you in this book's series of personalized, erotic talk sex-coaching sessions. Your wanton welfare comes down to what you want to make of it, and I'm here to make you as verbally voluptuous as you can be.

This Book Is For You

We're all sexual beings and we can all stand to learn a thing or two from employing some erotic talk, whether sweet, racy, hilarious, indecent, or perverse. I crafted this book for adults of all ages, of all sexual orientations, and in every kind of relationship. So when I use terms like *partner*, *lover*, *relationship*, and *couple*, know that I am referring to you and whomever you're eager to engage with erotically. As long as you're looking to experiment with and master all sorts of sex communication, from heart-to-heart sex talks to sinfully seductive confessionals, this book's for you. We can all learn from each other, including from the men and women whose sentiments and experiences are captured in my Erotic Talk Survey. Whether you're young or old, single or in a committed relationship, straight, gay, or bisexual, yours is the sex life I'm dedicated to improving through the tactful and titillating use of erotic talk.

How to Read This Book

Each chapter begins with objectives to aim for and ends with a part wrap-up, part self-evaluation check-in where you'll be asked to record things like your successes, highlights, challenges, future opportunities, thoughts, sensations, and emotions. We start our discussion of every topic by gauging where you're at and allowing you to reflect upon your desires. These topics, which include Rules of Engagement, are followed by an Erotic Talk Action Plan or exercises offering time guidelines, suggestions for lust-inducing locations, required materials, and peaking potential—though none of these elements are set in stone. Your peaking potential is gauged as:

1: Pulse-quickening
2: Automatically arousing
3: Seriously sexy reactions going on
4: Can-hardly-catch-my-breath climactic
5: Out-of-this-world orgasmic!

You're in charge, so if you want to linger longer or aim for a higher peak, you've got my full support.

Whether pursuing an action plan or exercise, don't allow yourself to feel rushed. Take your time, moving at a pace that feels right for you and your partner. Speaking of whom. . . . You may choose to read this book on your own and ask your partner to join you in certain exercises. Or you may want to read it together and compare notes. Either way, be prepared to expend some effort at various points. But that's the beauty of sex books: By work, we mean play!

A final note: Some couples may want to pick and choose their activities rather than follow an A-to-Z program approach. This may be especially true for those of you who feel confident that yours is a relationship that's already geared up for engaging in all sorts of erotic talk right away. You may be tempted to skip ahead, which is fine, but it never hurts to brush up on the fundamentals that can transform sexy talk from impaired to unimaginably hot.

1

Getting Ready for Erotic Talk: Building Trust and Communication

IN CHAPTER 1, YOU'LL LEARN HOW TO:

☑ Consider the wide variety of aural delights at your disposal.

☑ Judge whether your relationship is ready for sexy talk.

☑ Evaluate your erotic talk preferences.

☑ Feel out your erotic talk potential while getting things going at basic lingo levels.

☑ Get yourself and your partner in the know on the importance of true intimacy and positive sex communication.

"Erotic talk is huge —massive— a significant part of our sexual encounters, from role-playing to orgasm-inducing triggers. I like it when my partners are verbal during sex, which serves as validation that I'm turning them on." —Todd

Erotic Talk: Defining This Delectation

Hear the term *erotic talk*, and most people's minds are instantly flooded with sweaty sex scenes full of groaning, moaning, and trashy dirty talk.

The majority of sex books only fuel the stereotype that talking dirty is the only way to be sexually seductive with words, devoting a page or two max to the topic. Not much is said beyond encouraging the reader to surprise his or her lover with a nasty new "slip of the tongue." The consequence: Many lovers bite their tongue. Uncomfortable with dirty talk, or feeling that they can't compete with porn-star trash talk, they relegate erotic talk to "no go" territory. Incredible sex opportunities are missed.

In failing to deliver the bigger picture when it comes to hot, positive sex communication, these reads rob lovers of the chance to reach their full sexual potential. Talking sexy involves much more than blowing someone's mind with raunchy, loin-stirring sleaze. Your voice can be like molten chocolate, making your partner melt as you lay on the lust with lines like:

"I can hardly contain myself when I'm around you."

"Is that bulge in your pants for me?"

"You're all that I need, but I always want more of you."

"I'm feeling like quite the shameless exhibitionist right now. Wanna put on a show?"

Erotic talk encompasses many different forms of intimate communication. Don't worry, I'm not about to whip out my white sex-doctor coat (that's reserved for my own bedroom play) and rattle off some boring diatribe about the detailed intricacies of how humans transmit messages to one another in sexual, romantic relationships. But it's to your benefit to look at the many modes of lust-inducing language, from the romantic to the ravenous. Through music, poetry, pillow talk, and so much more, words have always been at the center of our passion playgrounds.

Verbal expression has the power to seduce when delivered the right way, to ignite our lusty imaginations as every word stimulates our biggest sex organ: the brain. Pleasure centers throughout the body come to life as we unearth and express our every sexual or romantic need, want, desire, and fantasy. Your voice becomes a provocative sexual instrument as you tease, demand, encourage, reassure, praise, satisfy, or surrender control to another.

So what are all of these modes of ammo-packed arousal? It's highly likely that you're already well aware of all of them, and an artist in at least one of the following. (Note: While the erotic weight of each category varies from person to person, I've rolled them out from the earthier to the sweeter to the raciest.)

Sex Talk: Perhaps the most heart-pounding of erotic talk, the purpose of a sex talk is to communicate with your partner about your sex life, sexuality, needs, wants, and desires. While these discussions can incorporate any of the other types of erotic talk, the objective is to check in with your lover, make a request, address an issue, share experiences or thoughts, negotiate sex acts, and more. It can be quite sexy to share each other's thoughts on myriad issues, like practicing safer sex, strategies for attaining orgasm, navigating a three-some, how to resolve a sexual disorder, and finding time for sex. A lot more than your ears perk up in talking about your sex life!

Affectionate Talk: "I think the world of you." "Nobody does that as well as you do." "I love your laugh." These tender exchanges express care, nurturance, support, and encouragement. Sometimes peppered with endearing pet names, like *babe* or *darling*, such sweet talk can be giddy, playful, flirty, and light while being complimentary, like "You look handsome in that tux, hot stuff." Silly or serious, it's hard not to be won over by the admirer's loving words and flattery.

Romantic Talk: "We are one. One flesh; to lose thee were to lose myself." Be still, my beating heart, John Milton. Who can resist declarations like this quote from a seventeenth century poem about the temptation of Adam and Eve? Such expressions build on affectionate talk by being more amorous and moving. They have a heroic, I-would-die-for-you quality, in which a love interest is often idealized. The person doing the wooing adds fuel to the flame with testaments like, "When I'm with you, the world ceases to exist," or "You are my soul mate." Such talk provides the ultimate erotic ego-stroke coupled with phrases like "I love you" and "I want all of you" that caress every fiber of our being, not just the sexual.

Spiritual Talk: Practiced in forms of sacred sex, like Tantra, that celebrate oneness with each other and the universe, these high-spirited energy exchanges are aimed at honoring your partner. This art of passionate awakening invites lovers to strip down to their sexual souls for some of the most intense sexual exchanges known to humankind. In having sex with spirit, lovers express respect and gratitude for each other and the Divine with greetings like, "I honor the divinity within you," or the Sanskrit "Namaste," which means "I bow to you." The whole being becomes involved, with lovers achieving a deeper sense of intimacy and bliss in what practitioners consider the ultimate in harmonious unions.

Sensual Talk: This kind of conversation indulges our erotic appetite by being more pleasure- and intimacy-oriented, more flirtatious, and focusing more on sex appeal. Lovers tap into their potential for greater physical and emotional intimacy by saying suggestive things like, "I've been wondering what else you can do with those lips," or "You'll have to forgive that I'm a little distracted. You seem to have me thinking about other unmentionable things. . . ." There is still a note of romance—for example, "I can't take my eyes off of you"—with lovers hinting that they want to touch, see, feel, smell, and taste more.

Seductive Talk: There is a fine line between the sensual and seductive, but here's the distinction between the two: Vivid, energetic, and even more suggestive than sensual talk, racy seductive talk leaves nothing to the imagination. Lovers stroke their carnal connection, erecting their eroticism by stating things like, "I'm about to get all over that spankable ass of yours," or "You have me so wet that it's trickling down my thighs." The goal here is more than attraction; lovers look to playfully articulate their sexual needs and desires: "I'm so swollen. What are you going to do about it?" Sometimes, it can take the form of an urgent demand: "I need to feel you deep inside of me now!"

Dirty Talk: Talking dirty is at the far end of the tame-to-hardcore spectrum of sexual expression. Lovers break out their sex-pistol selves with unrestrained, libidinal longings: "I could cum from watching you unload all over my tits" and "Get over here. I want your massive, raging beast slamming inside me." This approach can seem intimidating for some lovers, but others embrace it because it puts their sexual nature and desires out there clearly and emphatically. Listen to Oliver: "Both me and my girlfriend are turned on by hearing each other moan or talk dirty. It helps us to know what we want from each other and what's working while we are having sex. It helps us both explore areas of fantasies we might otherwise be afraid to try. Sharing is a way of slowly expanding and pushing limits—bringing fantasies from our private thoughts to the forefront of our relationship, and allowing us to share what we are sometimes embarrassed to mention."

Know that sexy talk can often fall into more than one of these categories, so don't get too hung up on them individually. Couples should feel free to change things up by using different styles to generate different sexual moods. Take Jaymes: "Talk is important to foreplay because it's more specific than touches or actions. While out somewhere, my girlfriend and I can whisper to each other things like 'I can't wait to hold you down and fuck you later.' That's much more vivid than a touch or kiss, and really lets you start getting excited about what's coming later."

In addition to all these efforts, it's only human to sexually express ourselves through the release of primal sounds. Sound alone captures our innermost, primitive sexual nature. Deep breathing, loud sighs, quick gasps, or the "earuptive" moans of orgasm—they're captivating and contagious.

Personally, I'm a screamer. When I'm with the right person in the right "space," with all the right moves and good energy, I can't help but release my internal state of ecstasy. The sexual experience is otherwise completely compromised if I try to hold it all in. Miranda can concur: "Verbal and vocal expressions are primal and show appreciation for my partner. My orgasms come from somewhere so deep, from my core. It's like it builds from my toes, the ends of my hair and my fingertips, and zaps into my core before it explodes from there. That guttural, one-breath scream that erupts just seems natural. How could I *not* have a magnificent orgasm if that sound is accompanying it?"

WHEN IT COMES TO FINDING the right pick-up line, humans are pretty easy. One magazine poll found that, in meeting someone, just saying hello will engage men 71 percent and women 100 percent of the time.

So get ready: This book is going to take you far beyond "talking dirty" tendencies to make sure you're on top of your game in everything the erotic talk arena has to offer your sex life. In this chapter, you'll learn how to be an irresistible flirt, a skillful romancer, a divine love deity, a dynamic seducer, and a riveting lover.

Do You Two Have the "Chops" for Erotic Talk?

Now that we've set the stage for different kinds of erotic talk, you may be dying to jump into the act with phrases ranging from "Bring that minx body of yours close to mine" to "I want your rock-hard cock in every warm, wanting hole of my aching body!"

But first, we need to find out where your relationship is when it comes to erotic talk, especially in its more sexually enticing forms.

Lovers are often frustrated or confused when their partner isn't receptive to talking sexy. As a result, people like Rashawn come to experts like me, bewildered and hurt that their lover isn't down with the teasing and temptations that go along with talking sexy: "Erotic talk just doesn't come naturally to either of us, and it sucks! At most, he'll say 'It was great' afterward, or 'It was nice,' or 'That was awesome.' But that's all we really get at, which is far from what those magazines say will happen if you take a Nike 'just do it' approach. Things don't happen that way. I just get shut down by him. If I ever commit to anyone else, we'll be very open in the sexy talk department from the start. I need what I'm willing to give."

Whether it's you, your partner, or both, sex communication in every form can be awkward and difficult. Most of us aren't taught how to be savvy with sex talk. Yet open lines of communication lead to an easier erotic connection and greater pleasure from foreplay to afterplay. They make you more orgasmic and improve the overall quality of your sex life and relationship. What's more, sex talks between lovers:

➜ Teach you about each other in a unique, wonderfully private way
➜ Relieve the anxiety of second-guessing each other's wants and levels of satisfaction
➜ Help you to steer clear of misunderstandings that can arise in seeking satisfaction
➜ Add excitement and decrease boredom in and out of the bedroom
➜ Build a level of meaningful intimacy
➜ Increase your feelings for each other, evoking compassion, love, desire, admiration, and a whole slew of other feel-good reactions
➜ Stoke the passion and magic
➜ Reignite the sexual spark for couples that have been together for a while
➜ Remove any sense of isolation or disconnect
➜ Boost monogamy

If this list of benefits doesn't propel you to embrace erotic talk for the sake of your sex life and your relationship, perhaps Sam can convince you: "If you can't tell your lover what you want, why are you rubbing mucous membranes with them? Telling someone what you want using erotic talk is the key to getting your needs met."

My sentiments exactly.

EROTIC TALK CHECKLIST

So let's examine whether your relationship is ready for erotic talk by considering any issues that may impact your ability as a pair to support each other in your passion talk pursuits. Answer the following yes/no questions:

→ Does your partner stay engaged when things get difficult or when you talk about how you feel about the relationship?

→ Is your partner willing to go the extra mile for you two to get to a place where you're better than ever?

→ Does your partner hold you in high regard?

→ Would you say that your partner comes to the erotic talk experience with an open mind?

→ Are you willing to create a safe space in which both of you can share freely?

→ Are you satisfied with the way you two communicate in general?

→ Are both of you willing to experiment with talking sexy?

→ Are you interested in what your partner has to say and vice versa?

→ Is it important to each of you to consider and try to satisfy the other's needs?

If you answered yes to most of these questions, congrats! You're ready for an erotic talk master class. Your relationship appears to have what it takes to succeed given the mutual respect, support, and friendship components that are vital to establishing and maintaining a rich and satisfying sex life.

If, however, you found yourself answering no to many of the questions, see if the following checklist better captures your relationship:

→ Do you or your lover share things in confidence only to have that information used against you later?

→ Is your lover preoccupied with himself or herself during sex?

→ Does your relationship tend to be one-sided in that just one partner's needs—in or out of the bedroom—are attended to?

→ Does your partner have a habit of putting you down during arguments or in day-to-day conversation?

→ Do you withhold certain things from your partner for fear that you'll be judged?

→ Does one partner tend to be critical while the other is withdrawn?

→ Does one partner usually blame the other for a failure to communicate and as the source of any relationship problems?

→ Is it difficult to persuade your partner to eroticize sex in any way?

→ Does your partner have trouble expressing him or her self sexually?

If you answered yes to most of these questions, you need to proceed with caution when it comes to erotic talk. You and your lover have barriers in your relationship that you'll need to overcome for this to be a rewarding, mutually satisfying, and safe experience.

Both of these checklists highlight elements that are critical to a successful and wildly fun experience with erotic talk. These include:

Ease of Communication: Are you and your partner effective communicators when it comes to discussing issues that have nothing to do with sex? Effective communicators are people who:

→ Express themselves clearly, honestly, and simply, while being mindful to resist saying things that are overly negative or irrelevant. For example, instead of saying, "This place is a mess because you won't take out the garbage," your partner might say, "If we want a clean home, I really need for you to help me out by taking out the garbage."

→ Don't jump to conclusions. For example, instead of responding to his partner's concerns about an outfit with, "So you think I'm a terrible dresser? Are you saying that I'm not attractive?" a man might attempt to understand his partner's comment by asking for more information, like "Is it that you don't like the shirt? The pants? Is it the color?"

→ Listen and confirm what is being said—for example, paraphrasing (rephrasing what you think is being said in your own words)—without getting defensive.

→ Validate. Even if they don't agree with what's being said, even if they think you're totally off your rocker, they tell you that they can understand where you're coming from. For example, your partner gives reassurances: "You're entitled to your feelings. I can't fault you for them."

→ Ask open-ended questions to learn more, including how to move forward on an issue. These are questions that get beyond one-word responses; it's about reaching a solution or seeing the bigger picture of what's being discussed.

→ Consider how nonverbals, like body positions and use of touch, impact what they're saying. Effective communicators are similarly tuned into what's being expressed by a lover's gesture, tone of voice, and body language.

→ Use positive reinforcement (praise) or constructive criticism (where they state what they like, followed by a suggestion for improvement) when responding to another's efforts.

They're never critical or judgmental when sharing takes place.

Trust: Trust is at the heart of two people interacting effectively and erotically. Trust is being comfortable with and relying on your partner's character, instincts, and truthfulness. Trust affects sexual relationships in terms of what you're able to talk about and the ease of communication. Erotic talk won't be pleasurable or gratifying without trust, including the trust that boundaries will be respected, that you're in this to make sex better for both of you, and that sharing will be mutual. Without trust, the sex can be pretty lousy, believe me.

I once had a lover who I couldn't completely trust with my heart, even during those times when he wanted it. Because he hurt me a number of times, I knew we had no business being together. This lack of trust and our terrible overall communication affected our abilities when we did get busy. Erotic talk of any kind, from whispering sweet nothings to basking in an aural afterglow, was out of the question because I didn't feel safe enough emotionally to give it a try. Learn from my mistake and make sure that you're giving yourself everything you deserve when it comes to sex communication, beginning with trust. While somebody may want to get all over your backside, if they're not watching your back, you end up getting screwed in more ways than one.

Equality: First, the power dynamics of the relationship should be such that lovers are on an equal playing field. If lovers disrespect each other by not seeing themselves as equals, it can have a toxic effect. Who, for example, wants to hear dirty talk like, "You're such a whore" when the words are used by his or her partner to put him or her down daily? Such statements aren't sexy when you consider their context. Second, both partners need to be on board for upping their intimacy—knowing that the objective is shared pleasure and satisfaction. The best sex involves a shared reaction where lovers feel like a team. Selfish lovers need not apply.

Closeness: Partners are more receptive to erotic talk when they feel close to each other, a feeling that usually develops over time and by sharing experiences. Many people have trouble being verbal and expressive unless they feel intimate with their lover, as is the case for Nate's partner: "My lover is introverted sexually. It is difficult for her to express herself, her wants, and desires. As we've gotten closer, we've been able to talk about sex more. Talking to her helps her see how freeing it can be. It helps her explore her own ability to vocalize her sexual thoughts, which is all very exciting to me."

These relationship essentials matter because you're about to get raw with each other, in the sense of exposing your deepest desires and needs. Most people are apprehensive when it comes to talking about sex and their relation-ship because stripping down to their sexual soul can feel risky and frighten-ing. The more you can count on your partner to be supportive, trustworthy, respectful, and open, while being playful and maintaining a sense of humor, the less risky and more stimulating your erotic talk experience will be. In turn, you'll be having the time of your life in the bedroom and beyond.

Erotic Talk Action Plan: Launching Your Sex Communication Campaign

Sexual interactions are like sporting events. They typically start with a warm-up (foreplay), followed by the main event (sex play), and end with a cool-down (afterplay). But what is rarely considered in this analogy is the training that gets the athletes ready for their match. Athletes always show up looking pumped and ready to rumble. We admire their chiseled forms and impressive pregame moves, but we often overlook what got them to the point where they're ready to perform: an awesome amount of effort.

Incredible sex, in many respects, follows the same path. Both individually and as a couple, lovers need to work out to reach their peak performance condition. What they get out of their sex sessions comes down to what they put into their practice—mind, body, and heart. In realizing the sex of our dreams, just like an athlete, we all need to work on our issues, perfect our techniques, and put serious thought into everything that can affect our ability to perform. It's a widespread misconception that, as sexual beings, we should automatically be good in bed—not true. But what is true is that we can all get there with the right attitude, guidance, and commitment to lots of toe-curling practice!

> **RESEARCH HAS FOUND** that the verbal reactions that shut down communication of any kind are criticizing someone's character, being defensive, stonewalling, and contempt. So beware!

So let's start at square one. What do you need to do to launch your erotic talk efforts?

1. Decide what you want out of talking sexy.
2. Sell positive sex communication to your partner.
3. Suspend judgment, set ground rules, and respect each other's boundaries.
4. Learn what not to say and what words you can use.

1. Decide What You Want Out of Talking Sexy

One of my favorite sex mantras is: You're responsible for your own sexual pleasuring. Too often, we put the responsibility of being sexually gratified on our partner's shoulders. Females, in particular, have been raised to think that men are responsible for their sexual pleasure, especially in helping them attain the coveted "Big O." The truth of the matter is that each of us is in charge of our own sexual satisfaction. Our ability to reach peak sexual responsiveness is within ourselves—not under our partner's control. Once you accept that truth, and articulate what you want out of sex, you're well on your way to realizing your just pleasure.

This starts with you focusing on what you want, beginning with the following Erotic Talk Preferences Quiz.

Using whole sentences or jotting down key words, respond to the following questions that ask you to consider your hopes, needs, and desires. Where multiple-choice answers are provided, feel free to check more than one if appropriate.

TIME: 15–20 minutes

LUST-INDUCING LOCATION: anywhere you can scribble your thoughts without someone looking over your shoulder (e.g., a quiet corner of a coffee shop)

MATERIALS: pencil (and a notebook if you don't want to write in the pages of this book)

PEAKING POTENTIAL: 1—although thinking about different sex topics and scenarios can stimulate a voracious appetite for more

A. I need to be in the following type of relationship to engage in erotic talk:
___ Stranger
___ Casual
___ Dating
___ Committed
___ Other: _____

B. The types of erotic talk I want to explore are:
___ Sex talk
___ Affectionate talk
___ Romantic talk
___ Spiritual talk
___ Sensual talk
___ Seductive talk
___ Dirty talk

C. I couldn't handle erotic talk that would be described as:
___ Degrading
___ Sappy
___ Cheesy
___ Deep/Profound
___ Hardcore

___ Graphic
___ Flirtatious
___ Emotional
___ Touchy-feely
___ Seductive
___ Other: _____

D. Words that are out of the question
include _____ .

E. Words that turn me on
include _____ .

F. Sex acts that I'd like to focus on
during erotic talk include:
___ Kissing
___ Caressing
___ Masturbation
___ Mutual masturbation
___ Hand job
___ Erotic massage
___ Fellatio (oral sex on a male)
___ Cunnilingus (oral sex on a female)
___ Analingus (oral-anal pleasuring)
___ Vaginal-penile intercourse

___ Anal sex
___ Titty fucking (pressing the breasts
around a phallus)
___ Gluteal sex (penis rubs butt crease)
___ Intefermoral sex (thrusting between
thighs)
___ Tantric exchanges
___ Sharing fantasies
___ Role-playing fantasies
___ Stripping
___ Using sex toys
___ Fetish play
___ Other: _____

G. Engaging in erotic talk would turn
me on during:
___ Foreplay
___ Main Sex
___ Afterplay
___ Commute to work
___ Working hours
___ Work breaks
___ A date
___ Other: _____

H. Sounds that turn me on during sex play include:

__ Heavy breathing
__ Groaning
__ Moaning
__ Silence
__ Music
__ Gasping
__ Screaming
__ Sighing
__ Wailing
__ Laughter
__ Crying for joy
__ Whimpering
__ Giggling
__ Other: _____

I. I am up for communicating about sex via:

__ Email
__ Text messaging
__ Instant messaging
__ Cybersex
__ Phone
__ Face to face

Don't get distressed if you're not sure how to answer some of these statements. It can be difficult to think about what you want—what you could possibly ask for and receive—when we're just getting started. While reading further, you may find that some answers change or reveal themselves. Consider revisiting the quiz later to see if your responses need tweaking.

2. Sell Positive Sex Communication to Your Partner

If talking sexy, or just talking about sex in general, is your idea, then it's your job to get your partner to sign on with you. The next time you and your lover are enjoying a private, relaxed moment, let your honey know that you're keen on exploring erotic talk, that it has your sex drive piqued. You might add, "I know this sounds like it's coming out of nowhere, so don't feel pressure to respond right away."

If your partner is intrigued—or at least listening—follow up with some key selling points about what positive sex communication can achieve, such as the following:

→ More delightfully risqué moments in a hotter, stronger relationship. Equally appealing: You'll know how to arouse, delight, and nourish each other in innovative ways.

→ A thriving relationship—one that's continually reinventing itself so it can evolve and grow—thanks to honest sex communication.

→ Playful, fun, turn-me-on moments.

→ New excitement and exploration from bringing wicked fantasies to life that can satisfy both of your physical and emotional needs.

If your lover is resistant or defensive, bring in irresistible reinforcements, explaining that:

→ Having sex takes on deeper meaning when underlying thoughts and feelings are erotically expressed.

→ Becoming effective communicators helps to avoid sexual dysfunction and to overcome such issues should they arise.

→ Lovemaking isn't mechanical when expressing and meeting each other's needs.

→ One-third of sexually satisfied couples admit they wish their sex life could be improved.

→ Declarations of love nourish the relationship.

→ Happy lovers are those in relationships marked by verbal kindness.

→ Talking about sex is an exhilarating exchange of sexual energy.

While you need to become a salesman making the right pitch, you've got the good fortune of knowing your target market most intimately. Take advantage. Instead of bombarding your lover with a slew of selling points, craft your persuasions around your particular goals and desires and what you think your partner is likely to respond to and able to be coaxed by. And as you delve into the topic, try to diffuse any concerns he or she may have. As mentioned, a lot of people will jump to the conclusion that what you're suggesting is nothing more than verbal smut. Even if that's your hope, you need to be sensitive to the possibility that your lover may need further encouragement to talk like two truckers in heat. Many people need to be coaxed out of their shell, either a little—or a lot. Reassure your lover that you have no interest in being demeaning, derogatory, or vile (unless, of course, that fits the bill).

More than anything, the point to emphasize is that you long to explore ways to share, play, appreciate, and bond with your partner while supercharging your sex life. You're curious about the types of sexy talk that have the potential to increase intimacy, arousal, and sparks. Finally, if your lover is still holding back, say that you want to see what all of the fuss is about after reading what so many erotic talk survey respondents had to offer:

"It definitely heats things up for him and relays my interest in what he is doing. I like when my partner is verbal during sex; it serves as validation that I'm turning him on."

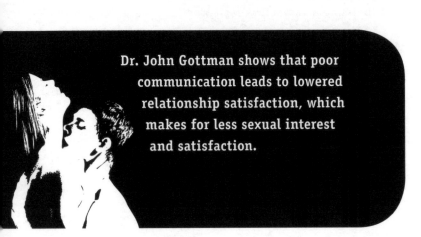

Dr. John Gottman shows that poor communication leads to lowered relationship satisfaction, which makes for less sexual interest and satisfaction.

"My opinion is this: You should always communicate what you want during sex. Whatever it is, even if it's negative, you can probably figure out a way to say it that won't kill the mood. Know your partner, choose your words carefully, but by all means say what you think."

"Any kind of erotic sounds and words always heighten the act."

"I couldn't imagine silent sex! Too much talking is usually a bad sign because it means one or both of the partners are insecure, but silence is *awkward*. Verbal communication, whether it's moans or dirty talk, is so important!"

"Couples only stand to benefit in communicating about sex in a favorable way. With sexual wisdom, you can only have a stronger, healthier relationship."

And leave it with one of my favorites, Rumi: "Each moment from all sides rushes to us the call to love. We are running to contemplate its vast green field. Do you want to come with us?"

Talk is sexy. And who better to talk it up with than you?

3. Suspend Judgment, Set Ground Rules, and Respect Each Other's Boundaries

You need to create a safe space, free of judgment and negativity, in which to share. Defined rules and mutually agreed upon boundaries encourage and support your every curiosity. Once you've established a welcoming, nurturing environment, you'll both feel free to share sexual wishes, generate greater intimacy, and increase the range and depth of your erotic conversations.

SUSPENDING JUDGMENT

Lovers need to suspend judgment if they are going to feel comfortable exposing themselves to each other. The quality of your sex only goes up when you allow for mutual trust and self-disclosure for heightened awareness and understanding. To establish a judgment-free zone for erotic talk:

➜ Don't put down or belittle your lover: "How was it? Truth be told, I've had better."

→ Don't make your lover feel wrong or dirty for expressing his or her wants or desires: "You want to lick my what? That's disgusting!"
→ Don't give suggestions for improvement immediately after sex: "No teeth next time, okay?"
→ Avoid reacting to your partner with demeaning labels: "I can't believe you did that. You pervert!"

Once you've agreed to avoid judging each other to invite self-disclosure, it's wise to set ground rules for talking about sex.

SETTING GROUND RULES

Couples who come up with guidelines for sharing and expressing themselves have a safe foundation on which to proceed with erotic experimentation. To help you draft your list of ground rules, I've provided some of the most popular guidelines my students have relied on over the years:

→ Everything that is shared remains confidential.
→ No personal attacks.
→ Be honest.
→ Respect and appreciate other opinions and values.
→ It's okay to ask.
→ Use "I" statements. (This is where you speak for yourself, owning your thoughts, feelings, needs, wishes, hopes, and experiences, instead of attributing them to others by using *you* or *we*.)
→ Withhold judgment.
→ Have fun!

On a piece of paper, write the rules you both want to guide your sexual discussions. As you draft your rules, consider the following tips in addition to those discussed earlier:

→ Don't tease, coerce, or embarrass the other person.
→ Be the real you.
→ Be attentive to equality. Some lovers can be overly expressive; this may be because they have found an effective way to get their lover's attention or to have greater influence on the relationship. While being dominant can be a total turn-on in the bedroom, neither lover should dominate sex talks.
→ Desire shouldn't be a demand. Lovers should not feel sexual pressure to engage in a behavior simply because the desire has been shared.
→ Don't feel obliged to tell all (e.g., past sexual history).
→ Be compassionate.

Once you've both agreed on your ground rules, feel free to call each other out on them when necessary. Even when lovers try their best to follow the rules, they may occasionally forget or break one. A gentle reminder of what was mutually agreed upon should do the trick.

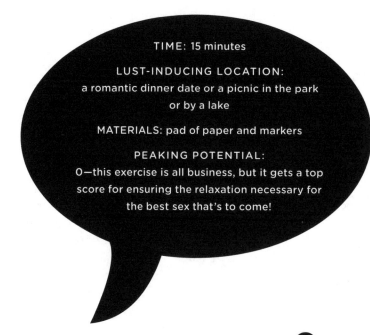

TIME: 15 minutes

LUST-INDUCING LOCATION:
a romantic dinner date or a picnic in the park or by a lake

MATERIALS: pad of paper and markers

PEAKING POTENTIAL:
0—this exercise is all business, but it gets a top score for ensuring the relaxation necessary for the best sex that's to come!

Respecting Boundaries

When it comes to something as personal as sex, it can't be overstated: Lovers need to understand and respect their partner's boundaries. You must establish "do not cross" lines when it comes to using certain words or vocalizing certain acts. As you sort through what gets a red light or green light, be prepared for some negotiating.

For example, consider the use of off-color or swear words. Depending on your partner's religious beliefs, saying something like "You're so god-damned sexy!" or "Jesus! I need to feel your pussy *now*!" may only earn you a slap in the face. Some people aren't into hearing their lover curse or use what's broadly considered offensive language, yet others get instantly aroused when their partner swears like a sailor, laying on the filth.

I can't stress it enough: What works for one person doesn't necessarily work for another, especially when it comes to talking smack. Preferences can also change over time, as Maria points out: "Sometimes, I want to be called a bitch, and other times I don't. I usually don't

like to use words like *cunt* because it sounds really, really dirty. So we'll save it for our naughtier encounters. I'm really lucky because we have such good communication. We talk about what will fly ahead of time."

No matter how well you think you know your partner, there may be times when he or she surprises you with what turns them on. Consider the following response I received as part of the Erotic Talk Survey: "The best talking dirty line so far in getting a reaction out of my lover is 'I hate you.' I don't know why. Maybe it's that it implies a taboo attraction that was so counter to what her rational brain wants, which is really arousing."

4. Learn What Not to Say and What Words You Can Use

If you're worried about saying the wrong thing, then having one or several conversations about what's acceptable and what's not should quell your concerns. Yet it's impossible to cover every detail and scenario, and you may inadvertently step on a land mine. To lower your risk, let's look at what not to say before going any further.

Dirty vs. Degrading

Erotic talk means different things to different people, and that includes what gets labeled *dirty* versus *degrading*. The impact of derogatory words like *bitch*, *slut*, *whore*, *bastard*, *fairy*, *queer*, or *nympho* depends on whom you're speaking to. Some people might find these words arousing in certain circumstances, while others might find them repulsive and utterly inappropriate at all times. This is what Alessa has to say: "*Slut* is an off-limits word. I've had guys try to talk dirty to me and use this word and it is a huge turn off."

Other people, like Tava, find certain words better than others, though it's not always obvious why: "I would never be okay with being called a bitch or a whore, but for some reason I'm fine with being called a slut or a brat. The first two terms are probably much more socially stigmatized for me, while slut has kind of been reclaimed by feminists and brat implies a childish playfulness in the bedroom."

The same goes for talking about certain acts, as Rich learned the hard way: "My wife and I were having sex and we were involved in a little anal stimulation (me using my finger on her anal opening) and she was into it until I said, 'Oh yeah, baby, I'd like to fuck your ass,' and she stopped and was like, 'That's *never* gonna happen.' Talk about an instant downer!"

Work toward an understanding that words are never meant to demean or insult but to heat up and play up the moment. As long as lovers are secure in knowing that certain words are to be used solely in the context of sex play, they can feel empowered to really spice things up.

Don't Even Think About It: What Not to Say

"Ooo yeah, baby. Give it to me. Ooo. That's right. Aww yeah, come to mama, big daddy. Yeah, right there. . . ." When it comes to talking sexy, porn clichés are a dime a dozen. Couples might have a good time making fun of porn, especially if they indulge in a fantasy that they are adult film stars, with lines like "Give it to me, big boy," "Suck it, baby, yeah, that's right," or "Yes—harder, deeper, harder!" But for most people, the language used in porn flicks doesn't fly. According to Manuel, it comes off as insincere and contrived: "A running dialogue like some cheesy porn movie is sort of a turn-off. Talking sexy always has to be genuine. Anything fake is a big no-no."

Another verbal violation is going the medical route. While terms like phallus, vulva, penis, and vagina work when you're in an academic setting, talking to a healthcare provider about sex, or having a parent-child talk about the birds and the bees, they can ruin the mood in sexual relationships. Some people are comfortable using formal language, like "I can't wait to get all over your erect penis," but the vast majority don't find it the least bit stimulating. At the other end of the spectrum, there are many informal, slang terms for the genitals that belong in high-school locker rooms—not in the bedroom. The following is a list of the worst offenders for penis:

arrow	magic wand
beefstick	mighty scabbard
chubby	pecker
dinger	salami
dip stick	sphincter-lizard
dong	sword
dork	tally-whacker
flesh kabob	torpedo
gun	trouser trout
hog	tube steak
Johnson	wang
little Elvis	wiener
longhorn	worm

I could go on, but you probably get the point. Unfortunately, when it comes to the ladies, I'm afraid it doesn't get any better. Words that will make a guy sound like he's been watching too much *Beavis and Butt-Head* and should therefore be avoided at all costs in referring to a woman's sex organs include:

bearded clam	snapper
bleed hole	snatch
buttered muffin	spear
fur burger	tattlemouse
gash	trap
jive	tuna taco
lickety-slit	tunnel of love
love tunnel	vertical smile
mock orange	whisker biscuit
secret garden	

Saying any of these can immediately lead to game over, as Penny confirms: "We have no rules, though he knows that if he ever mentions 'the shocker' that my entire pelvic area will clamp down tighter than a frog's behind."

Words You Can Use

Having considered some of the worst offenders, which you may or may not agree with, let's shift our discussion to words you *can* say. In talking to people about their sexual vocabulary over the years, I've found that tastes vary widely. So while the following words get a green light from a large number of people, your lover might conclude that they are ridiculous, offensive, a turn-off, or all three. Personally, *cunt* has always been an abhorrent word to me, but some women feel empowered when they claim a term that has been used to degrade women. Before adopting these words, then, make sure to talk to your lover about which ones work for you and under what circumstances.

When it comes to describing a woman's vulva or vagina, lovers may use:

beaver	muff
box	muffin
chalice	pussy
coochie	slit
cooter	snatch
crotch	twat
cunt	vajayjay
hole	

Mound relates to the area over a woman's pubic bone, and bush refers to her pubic hair. Cherry, sacred spot, and love button are words for her clitoris.

For a man's penis and scrotum, partners may like:

balls	lingam
beast	love muscle
boner	member
bulge	nuts
cock	pecker
hard on	prick
it	rod
jade stalk	shaft
jewels	skin flute
joystick	tool

HUMANS HAVE HAD a lot of free time on their hands given that the number of terms for masturbation run into the hundreds. Sadly, the vast majority are nowhere near sexy, like *slap your noodle* and *tuna tickle*.

Be careful with names for penis that are a real guy's name. We've all known people named Dick, Peter, Willy, Jimmy, or Woody, and probably don't think about these words in a sexy context (especially if the "Dick" in question is someone's dad).

Words that refer to a woman's chest should be considered as well. Most in this category are total boobs (pun intended). Many will make you sound like an *Animal House* frat boy:

boulders	jugs
gazongas	knockers
headlights	melons
hooters	rack

That's not to say, however, that lovers can't have fun with words like these and others, but *tits*, *bosom*, and *bust* are the more common go-to terms.

When it comes to the buttocks, most words tend to work, though you and your lover should talk it out if either of you has an issue with any of the following:

arse	cheeks
ass	derriere
backside	rear
booty	rump
bottom	tail
bum	tush
buns	

The anal opening is typically called *asshole*, *back door*, or *butthole*.

Since it's possible that you completely disagree with me on these word lists, I've crafted the following exercise so you can call the shots.

Discuss all the words you like and don't like for female genitalia, male genitalia, vaginal-penile sex, anal sex, masturbation, male and female ejaculation, fellatio, cunnilingus . . . any category of words you could see yourselves touching upon at one point or another during sex play.

Come to an agreement on which words make your "banned" list, taking time to explain why (beyond the fact that they sound dumb or juvenile). Let your lover know which words you find sexiest and in what circumstances.

Just getting the words out there increases one's comfort level with sexual terminology. Discuss with your partner personal nicknames or loving terms, like sugar stick, love dart, or Mr. Happy for him, or flower, blossom, or love petals for her.

TIME: 30 minutes

LUST-INDUCING LOCATION:
your TV room couch

MATERIALS: none

PEAKING POTENTIAL: 0.75—the mental images that come with some words can get you thinking about a lot more than this exercise

Why You Don't Want to Respond the Wrong Way

Even when couples thoughtfully map out their likes and dislikes, one partner, in the throes of passion, may take a chance and throw something out there that ruins the moment. It's also conceivable that a lover may accidentally mutter a banned term or try something that makes the other person recoil. Remember Rich? He's the guy who got caught up in the action and told his wife, "I'd like to fuck your ass," and it killed the moment. If your partner slips up, there are two ways to react:

1. Take a deep breath and make a mental note to address the comment later. Then let it go and refocus on your pleasuring without getting worked up. (Note, however, that if you get more reactive in your pleasuring, your partner might misinterpret your nonverbal body language as affirmation for what he or she said.)

2. Play with the comment, steering the dialogue back to what you like. Rich's wife would have done better with a coy response such as, "Baby, you know I'm not that type of girl. But I'd love to know what you're gonna to do for me if I even consider doing something that nasty." Assuming Rich and his wife discussed their boundaries and know the rules of erotic talk, he should not mistake this comment as an actual promise. He should have fun batting the ball back and forth with her, explaining the many ways he's good at getting her all smutty.

More than anything, don't give your lover a hard time if this happens, especially if he or she gets the message quickly. As Leonard Cohen once said, "There is a crack in everything. That's how the light gets in." It's not always bad to test one's boundaries, as Campbell can attest: "I've found my boundaries have expanded over time. I suppose there are some words and phrases that I have not heard, but for the most part I am not offended if the language turns hard sometimes. 'You're a dirty whore' has turned me on more than once, but it's not for everyday use. I've not had to say 'Don't say that' yet."

Now, should you be the one who slips up, hopefully your lover will be as gracious as you. If you find that you've dropped a booty bombshell, don't make a big deal about it. Just get yourself back on track, perhaps making up for it with loving sentiments, including affectionate physical gestures like sprinkling your lover's face with kisses. Then later, once you've both recouped from ravishing each other, take a moment to apologize. Keep it simple: "I'm sorry that I said XX. I got carried away in the moment." Provide other reassurances, if necessary, and then promise not to set off such aural artillery again. Both of you should agree to a truce. After all, you're in this for the same reason: to make love (not war) for the hippiest, trippiest sex.

Chapter 1 Check-In

Now that you have a better sense of what you want and what your partner may be up for, ask yourself the following questions:

1. Which goals are appropriate, given the type of relationship you have?
2. Which goals are achievable at this time?
3. How can you take the next steps toward these goals?

To consider the possibilities available to you and your lover, read on: The following queries may help you fashion a game plan whenever you sense apathy or resistance from your partner.

Do you become easily deterred by your lover's inability to engage you? You can have what you want to a certain degree if you don't let your lover throw you off course. You can take matters into your own hands, pulling the load for both of you, as Micah has: "I have had a partner for two years who is silent during sex. This is because of his upbringing, and he has become so conditioned to it from other lovers that I don't think he'll break his habits. I, on the other hand, make noise, despite the neighbors. I am also really good at telling my partner what does and doesn't feel good. If I allow myself to be discouraged by his silence, then I fear not getting what I want and need, including hearing my response."

Can you act as a source of support for your lover? Erotic talk isn't going to come easily to all partners, even those who are willing. Your efforts will be more successful if you can be a source of strength, like Kendal's partner: "My lover is so encouraging, knowing it's hard for me to make noise. The more I talk or moan, the more excited he gets. I started getting into erotic talk more for him, but I find that it helps me feel more into the moment when I play everything up a little."

Can you accept your partner where he or she is at? Always accept and respect your partner's comfort level. Some lovers are up for erotic talk and possess a great deal of potential,

but it can take time, understanding, and gentle encouragement from you to help them reach new heights. Consider what Charles has to say: "For me, erotic talk is communicating my sexuality to my partner. It's simple love and affection, like 'You're cute.' " That is indeed cute, but something tells me that with the right set of circumstances, Charles could be talked into a bit more.

In this chapter, you may have found that you and your partner are up for a whole lot more than you anticipated— or that you have much more erotic talk at the tip of your tongue than you realized. We've hit on all of the different ways you can sex things up with what you say. We've evaluated your preferences and explored your potential for broaching the topic. We've established boundaries, identified appropriate language, and set rules. We're well on the way to making things sensational in synchronizing these seduction strategies. So let's move on to tackling some effective and oh-so-erotic talking tricks.

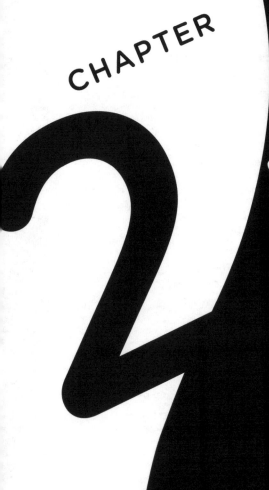

CHAPTER

2

"Coming" into Your Own with Erotic Talk:
Discover What Turns You On

IN CHAPTER 2, YOU'LL LEARN HOW TO:

☞ Overcome fear, self-doubt, and embarrassment issues.

☞ Master the art of erotic talk.

☞ Discover sources of unbridled inspiration.

☞ Feel confident and sexy by warming up your vocal chords.

☞ Get empowered by talking sexy while masturbating.

Whether you're hoping
to light a fire within, supercharge sex, or invite emotional release, the intrinsic power of your voice should never be underestimated. Chapter 2 is about you and your eroticism. This part of the book is all about self-discovery as you prime yourself for passion galore, starting with fantasy-provoking private time packed with exercises that focus on you, your voice box, and your abilities to talk sexily. We'll also explore ways that you can find your voice while dousing any concerns you have about getting loud. I want you to be comfortable with every type of erotic talk out there by the time we throw you into the ring so you'll be ready to bowl your beau over with debauchery in chapter 6.

ONE OF THE BIGGEST BARRIERS to experimenting with sexy talk is self-doubt. People often lack confidence when it comes to uttering the erotic, worrying they'll be bad at it. They seem to think that talking sexy requires being a smooth operator. Although an assured delivery can be impressive, erotic talk doesn't have to be—nor should it be—like listening to a polished performer. In fact, a large part of the charm and fun of erotic talk is the lightheartedness and personal effort you bring to it. Still, lovers put a lot of pressure on themselves to do things "right," refraining from trying something new if they're afraid they'll stumble or look foolish.

Never forget that there's no precise way to talk sexy. It's entirely and beautifully individual, and your personality and style are what will make your approach utterly unique and irresistible. If somebody is looking for a professional erotic talker, they can call one and pay for the privilege. But once you develop the right mind-set and start to recognize which words, phrases, and sounds work for you, chances are they will work wonders for your lover, who will be turned on and swept away by your sexpot self-assuredness.

Curing Your Verbal Performance Anxiety

Everyone knows about performance anxiety. It can happen on the stage or in the sack and be completely disabling. When this crippling fear of failure occurs during sex, the pressure to perform is so great that it can bring about the very failure that is feared.

Many people experience the same paralyzing fears and anxieties when it comes to erotic talk—a stage fright of sorts. People worry: What if I sound stupid? What if she doesn't think it's sexy? What if he's unimpressed? What if talking makes having sex harder instead of hotter? In this section, we take on all of these worries and more.

I'm uncomfortable with talking sexy. Whether it's because you're shy or your upbringing taught you that talking about sex is inappropriate, it's perfectly natural to feel uncomfortable if erotic talk is new to you. But don't let your inhibitions—or someone else's—keep you from giving it a try. In fact, holding yourself back probably contributes to your feelings of discomfort. So go ahead and give yourself permission to experiment. Experimentation is the first step toward discovery, and you may discover just how natural—and exciting—talking dirty can be. Stella didn't start talking sexy until she was well into middle-age: "It never came naturally for me to start using erotic talk with someone. But I decided to choose and say things that I never had before in order to enhance my sexuality. I had never said the word 'clit' out loud until I was forty-eight! Don't wait so long to be verbally explicit. I'm having the best sex of my life and communicating what I need, how I'm feeling, or what I'd like to do to my lover's gorgeous, hot body. It is so much fun!"

And if you feel uncomfortable with erotic talk because you're a parent, remember: Don't let family obligations keep you from staying in tune with your sensual self and your commitment to nurturing your sex life. Happy lovers make happier parents, so it's for your family's greater good if you let yourself get frisky and a little naughty on occasion. This kind of sexual self-care yields nothing but benefits to you, your career, your health, your family, and your emotional and spiritual development—not to mention your romantic life and sexual intimacy with your partner.

In fact, the need for balance can be a powerful motivator for parents to talk about sex. Listen to what Corey has to say: "We talk about sex pretty often. We have kids, so it helps to discuss it—otherwise you get overrun by other stuff and it's hard to get together on the whens and wheres. Erotic talk helps to make those moments happen as scheduled. The need for balance opens the door in being able to discuss other things."

I'm having trouble getting into the idea of erotic talk in general. Talking sexy isn't arousing for every-body. This is what Jordan has to say: "Mostly, it's that I don't always get turned on by it. Sometimes it comes off as cartoonish and can make me feel less connected to my partner. I'm more visual and tactile about sex, and the verbal stuff doesn't always do much for me."

A partner's willingness to indulge a lover's fancy is admirable. Such erotic bartering takes place in every sexual relationship to a certain extent, and if approached in the right way, both parties see returns on their investments quite quickly.

Say your partner is way into talking sexy but the idea doesn't do much for you. Well, before you back off, think of it this way: Being able to arouse somebody can be a total—and totally gratifying—head trip. When you utter sexy thoughts aloud, your lover becomes putty in your hands. You are the screen-writer and director of your private sex show, and you can develop the plot in whatever direction you'd like. So even if you're not into romantic innuendos or dirty talk, you may be surprised to discover how arousing it can be to have command of the situation. You just have to let yourself go there.

I'm not always in the mood for talking sexy. There is absolutely no reason to put pressure on you and your partner to always engage in erotic talk. Any activity can lose its thrill if you do it all the time. From the tame to the hardcore, nonstop erotic talk can become too much of a good thing— the same holds true for any sex act or sexual enhancer that starts to feel overused. You and your partner need to become adept at gauging what the mood calls for and then go with that. Maybe talking sexy isn't what you're craving, so go ahead and wrap yourselves in silence or enjoy the sounds of rustling sheets or the friction of sweaty bodies rubbing together.

What if my partner doesn't like what comes out of my mouth? Don't waste your energy speculating on what might happen. And definitely don't allow yourself to get consumed with self-deprecating thoughts; they don't do anybody any good, and they can throw up all sorts of pointless roadblocks. A kind lover and a good partner is one who will appreciate you for making the effort to juice up your sex life. (A partner who doesn't isn't worth your efforts, right?) If erotic talk is new territory for you, your lover will know that it's not easy and should be supportive and appreciative, not critical. This is what Mark had to say: "My lover is pretty shy and reserved, so it really gets me going when she talks about wanting me, needing me inside her, asking me to cum for her. When she vocalizes her rare desires for me to take her or use her (not in a degrading sense, but to be taken firmly as if I'm not to be denied), it drives me wild."

What if I run out of things to say? With all the inspirational resources available at your fingertips, you should have an abundant supply of lines, stories, and descriptors to use. That said, we don't want you sounding like a broken record. Lovers can get lazy and start relying on the same scenarios again and again. I am reminded of a lover whose erotic talk about spanking started to feel like beating a dead horse. At first, I loved it and it got my motor going, but after a while, my engine ran out of fuel when all it got was the same sexy talk—that didn't seem sexy anymore. Our erotic talk needed a fresh power source.

Just like any writer or entertainer, you need to constantly create new material. You've heard it before: Variety is the spice of life, particularly when it comes to action in the bedroom. Lovers need to switch things up, as Jake advises: "Certain phrases are golden, but the flip side is that these same phrases, repeated over and over again for years, become trite, expected, and lame. Get some new mojo every now and then!"

It's also important to realize that your sexual tastes and preferences evolve over time. What was sexy in your twenties may seem juvenile when you're older. What shocked you years ago may seem less shocking—and

more tantalizing—now. The way you use erotic talk can change as well, as Kerry explains: "Now that I'm more mature (and in a committed relationship), erotic talk has evolved from innuendo, double entendres, and sometimes overt flirting, to dirty talk in the sack! Sexy talk used to be a way to snag a guy or entice him into pursuit, but now it's a way to turn on my man (and vice versa), get him ultra horny in bed (and vice versa), or bring about an extra intense orgasm. It's about being more comfortable with myself, my sexuality, and our relationship. And I think the same holds true for him."

Whether it's a question of style or confidence in your abilities, your erotic talk will and should change over time. Lazara shares her experience: "I'm much louder now than I ever was during my sexually active college years. I'm a heavy panter and screamer now, for example, but that may be the result of not living in a dorm or in an apartment with roommates. I do say more of what I want, like 'Suck on my clit,' during the act, though not necessarily before it.

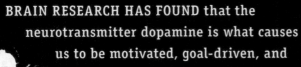

BRAIN RESEARCH HAS FOUND that the neurotransmitter dopamine is what causes us to be motivated, goal-driven, and focused when it comes to a love object. Your erotic talk efforts are one way to keep levels of dopamine elevated in the brain, driving "mad for you" reactions.

I am also now better at saying when something's not working, like 'We need lube,' or 'That position is uncomfortable.' "

I'm worried about juggling verbal and nonverbal at the same time. Sex plus erotic talk can feel like multitasking, and it's easy to get distracted with what you're doing instead of enjoying what's going on. If this happens, close your eyes, breathe deeply, and focus on what's happening in the moment. For example, if you're saying, "I want to feel your cock between my thighs" while giving your lover a hand job, say the words as you feel your lover's penis. Allow yourself to relish the moment by adding, "But I want to play with you a little bit first." Really focus on his penis— its weight, its texture, its shape, its hardness. Concentrating on what's before you frees you from the mental struggle of attempting two things at once. You can do this by keeping your focus on describing the senses being stimulated by the activity at hand. You can then remind yourself of your initial desire in saying "I am soooo close to feeling your hard on," "As soon as I get on you, you're so going to explode," or "My thighs can't wait to flex around your shaft."

I'm having trouble getting past the power certain words have over me. Words can be very powerful, especially when they've been used to suppress or to degrade. If a word exerts power over you, start by looking it up and studying its origin. Consider a word like *pussy*. Today, it may be used to put down a man as weak, effeminate, or cowardly, but *pussy* is thought to originally come from the Low German *puse*, meaning *vulva* or female *pudenda*, or possibly the Old Norse *puss* for *pocket* or *pouch*. So while *pussy* is often used as a crude way to refer to a female's genitals, it started out as no more than a medical term.

Another way to take control of the effect certain words have over you is to look at how they're used in other languages. The British use *fuck* without so much as a thought but *shag*—an old English word that means *matted, nappy hair*—provokes a stronger reaction. To the British, saying *shag* in the colloquial sense to mean sexual intercourse is the equivalent of using *fuck* in the United States. Here in the United States, it's quite different: *Shag* seems quaint and comical compared with *fuck*. So if you're an American who has trouble saying "Fuck me," for example, just remember that it's no big deal in the United Kingdom. If you're still having trouble, use a milder form of the same word, or learn how to say what you want in another language. Pick up a book of foreign phrases, and you'll be spouting fun and flirty phrases that will help you shed your inhibitions: In German, *Ich habe drei Eingange* means "I have three ports of entry," and *C'est une banane dans ta poche ou tu es juste content de me voir?* is French for "Is that a banana in your pocket or are you just pleased to see me?"

SPIRITUALITY MAY NOT BE the only reason people find themselves drawn to the study of Kabbalah. The Jewish mystical tradition regards the power of vowels as divine. Given that Madonna, the world's most successful female musician, has crooned more than her fair share of "ooo's" and "aahh's," it's no wonder she reached rock star deity status.

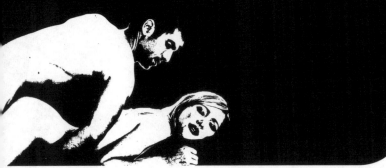

1. Make a list of the "dirty" words you're having trouble with.
2. Research the origins of the words on your list (some of which can be found using online dictionaries). Most likely, you'll discover that the words simply refer to body parts or "normal" activities, giving you the reassurance you need in knowing that a word's original meaning was perfectly innocent.
3. Practice using these words to desensitize yourself and strip them of their power to make you flinch. The more we say something, the less we fear it, and the less it is able to make us feel anxious or uncomfortable.

TIME: depends on how many words you want to look up.

LUST-INDUCING LOCATION: in the library, in front of your computer, or anywhere you can sit comfortably with a dictionary

MATERIALS: any word resource, such as a dictionary

PEAKING POTENTIAL: 0—sorry, this exercise is more scholarly than sexy, but you may have a different experience if words turn you on

Getting Inspired!

Most people are like Jade, who enjoys using different types of erotic talk: "I'm into a whole range. Depending on the mood, he turns me on when he says things like 'You're so beautiful' (if I know he means it), 'You're such a good lover,' 'That feels wonderful,' 'Oh, baby,' 'Oh, mama.' Dirty things are also a turn-on since they let me know he's into me and the sex, saying things like 'I'm about to blow my load,' or dirty things like 'You're such a sweet slut,' 'You're my little fuck toy,' or 'You love what I'm doing to your pussy, don't you?' "

And some know their favorites and are easy to please, like Dean: "I like 'Fuck me'—it's simple yet effective! I tend to like it more short and dirty. A few phrases here and there."

This section serves as your go-to guide for tuning into your sexy sense of self when it comes to affectionate, romantic, spiritual, sensual, seductive, and dirty talk. Here, you'll see which categories turn you on—and learn about resources offering shots of inspiration when your creative flair is waning.

You may have more untapped erotic energy than you realize, and we want to find that energy in strengthening your sexy talk abilities. The more you get in touch with your sensual essence, the more you'll discover about your capabilities, desires, fantasies, thoughts, and emotions—and how to express and act on them for greater allure and intimacy.

RESEARCH SHOWS THAT couples who are dating are more affectionate than those who are married. They're likelier to say things like "I love you" or "You're my best friend" than those who have tied the knot, and to express more nonverbal affection, like hugging, kissing, and holding hands. So if you've been committed for a while, make sure you express how much you mean to each other!

Just be sure to keep an open mind. You may surprise yourself when it comes to what turns you on. You may learn that an enchanting utterance can have you—or your lover—craving sex in a most unimaginable, exhilarating kind of way. So give yourself at least a taste of each type of sexy talk: You never know which ones will leave you feeling frisky and fresh for one another—and making some of your most primitive, passionate sounds.

YOU-MATTER-TO-ME INSPIRATION

Novelist and poet Josiah Gilbert Holland was right when he said, "The choicest thing this world has for a man is affection." People have long recognized that affection is a fundamental human need, and an exquisite one at that.

Affectionate inspiration is everywhere. Just walk into a card shop and you'll find an array of wholesome or cutesy, albeit sometimes nauseating, ways to tell someone you care about him or her. There are also a number of books out there, filled with loving testaments for those nearest and dearest to us, including our partners. These books show up in full force around Valentine's Day, but you can also find similar books year-round in the literature and romance sections of your local bookstore. Take your time to discover what resonates with you when it comes to expressing your fondness for your lover. No matter where your search takes you, you'll uncover seemingly endless ways to use words to draw in the object of your affection. Here are just a few:

➜ You look especially gorgeous today.
➜ I want to spend more time with you.
➜ I really miss you.
➜ We make a really nice couple, don't we?
➜ I need a hug from you.
➜ Can we do something special this weekend?
➜ I'm sorry that I've been preoccupied lately. You deserve more from me.
➜ We look good together.

When expressing thoughts like these, be careful not to overdo it. It's important that these sentiments sound and are actually genuine, especially in newer relationships, where declarations of affection can sometimes cause one party to retreat. Lovers who are just getting to know each other might find themselves thinking, *Does she really mean that? Is he just saying that to sleep with me?*

Showing your affection for another person can sometimes just be using a term of endearment that has special meaning, such as the following:

angel	lovey
babe	sugar
baby	sweetheart
darling	sweetie pie
honey	sweetness
love	sweet pea

Terms of endearment work with people like Meg: "I love that my husband calls me 'my sweetheart' and 'dear.' They just seem old-fashioned to me, and therefore more precious." The list of possible affectionate terms is endless, especially if you branch out to foreign languages. In Spanish, *Te adoro, mi amor* means "I adore you, my love." Or go with the Italian *cucciola mia* for "my pet," which literally translates to "my little animal," adding a whole other primal element to the bedroom. It goes without saying, of course, that you can and should come up with your own special nicknames for your beloved. One partner hooked me by calling me "sunshine," but randomly called me "bubbles" once, and that remained in the mix of loving lingo.

If it's difficult for you to come out and say affectionate things—or if you'd like to enhance your verbal efforts—consider writing secret messages and leaving them in places your lover will find them, like in his lunch bag, in her favorite shoes, or on his pillow. Small gestures like these are well worth the effort because affection is a primary way we form, maintain, and improve the quality of our relationships. Affection has also been shown to boost our mental and physical health by warding off loneliness and depression. It forms and transforms relationships, getting you both more of what you want. People never tire of having their significant other praise them and make them feel valued. Take Tess, for example: "My husband is so wonderful with appreciation and praise of me as a mother, wife, and lover—it makes me feel so loved."

HOT-AND-BOTHERED INSPIRATION

The Greeks called romantic love "madness of the Gods," and there's evidence of this insanity everywhere from poetry to cards and song lyrics. In fixating on their love object, people become consumed by a head-over-heels, feverish infatuation. Check out this letter written in the late 1800s by New Orleans lawyer Albert Janin to his girlfriend: "I cannot have a separate existence from you. I breathe by you; I live by you."

Those who aren't instantly blinded by love may experience a more gradual adoration and captivation that is shaped by time, intimacy, and shared life experiences. Their feelings—and the memories of what kindled the romance—are no less intense and can last forever.

I wanted you
That day at the beach
Because you were different
And because you smiled
And because I knew your world
was different.

— Rod McKuen

Stanyan Street & Other Sorrows

You could spend the rest of your days reading up on the limitless sources of romantic love—seems we humans simply can't get enough of it. But finding what works to guide your romantic talk efforts could take just a split second: Eyeball your music collection, and you may find lyrics that say it all. Or you may decide to spend more time, searching through literature (historical, fantasy, futuristic, collections, and even vampire, for example), music, and art for what captures "romance" for you.

To get you started, though, check out works by some of these romantic heavyweights: King Solomon's *Song of Songs*, Shakespeare's love sonnets, and the poetry of Sappho, William Blake, Walt Whitman, e. e. cummings, W. B. Yeats, Ralph Waldo Emerson, and Emily Dickinson. Lose yourself in a bookstore for an afternoon—you're sure to come out feeling flushed and informed.

When looking to romance your lover, just like we covered in our discussion of terms of endearment, don't restrict yourself to the English language. After all, there are several "romance" languages that have a lot to offer on the subject. There's the French phrase *faire la bouche en coeur*, which means "to flirt, or play coy" (the literal translation is "to make your mouth into a heart"). I'm a sucker for anything French, and *mon coeur est à toi* (my heart is yours) if you court me in that language. But you need to find out what appeals to you and your lover. Rest assured, just as people fall in love all over the world, there's a way to say it in every language:

The Russian expression for "love at first sight," *Ya vlubilsya bez oglyadki* (pronounced *yah vlyoo-BEEL-suh biz ah-GLYAHT-kee*) literally means "I fell in love without looking back."

The Romanian *mi-a r˘amas sufletul la tine* (pronounced *mee-ah ruh-MAHSS SOO-fleh-tool lah TEE-neh*), used to describe the feeling of falling in love, means "my soul is with you."

The German *ich hab mich in dich vernarrt* (pronounced *ikh hab mikh in dikh fer-NAHRT*) means "I'm crazy about you."

And again, like we discussed with terms of endearment, you can also keep things sweet and simple in delivering the occasional love note, like this fifteenth century musing from *The Nut-Brown Maid*: "For in my mind, of all mankind, I love but you alone."

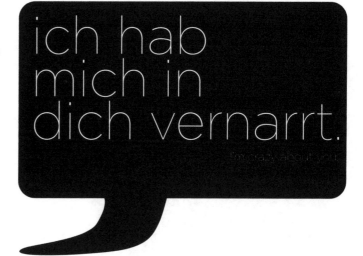

The poet John Keats once wrote in a private letter, "I could die for you. My Creed is Love and you are its only tenet . . . My love is selfish. I cannot breathe without you." The emperor Napoleon wrote passionate professions to his beloved Josephine: "A thousand kisses on your eyes, your lips, your tongue, your heart. Most charming of thy sex, what is thy power over me?"

Don't let this prose intimidate you—after all, these men lived at a time when romance was an art form. By contrast, sometimes it seems the best we get in the romance department these days is overly commercialized chocolates and roses on Valentine's Day. By simply choosing to value, exalt, and express romance in your life and in your relationship, you've taken a huge step forward.

1. As you think about composing a letter to your partner, remember that you want to speak from the heart. Let your feelings be your guide.
2. Begin with a loving salutation, like "My dearest . . ."

TIME: whenever the spirit moves you

LUST-INDUCING LOCATION: wherever you feel inspired

MATERIALS: pen and paper or laptop (although a handwritten effort is usually more endearing and visually appealing)

PEAKING POTENTIAL: 5—after all, love is the ultimate elixir

3. Ask yourself: When it comes to my lover, what do I appreciate? When it comes to our love, what do I want to celebrate? Then, let your stream of consciousness flow, playing up all of the qualities you love about this person, your relationship, and how you're moved by it all.

4. If you choose to make reference to the physical at any point, stick with kisses, caresses, hand-holding, gentle touches, etc., and stay elusive about the body parts you're thinking about.

5. Close with something personal, like "Yours forever . . ."

6. Mail your final copy (rather than email or hand delivery).

"Yours forever..."

"My dearest..."

SPIRITUAL INSPIRATION

I hesitate somewhat to use the term spiritual because many people interpret it to mean "religious." So just to clarify, when I say "spiritual," I'm getting at lovers relating to their inner spirits and a universal divine spirit. For some, however, the experience may in fact be religious and worshipping their God is an integral part of lovemaking, and that's fine if that's what works for them.

RESEARCH HAS FOUND that women, thanks to the media, envision romance as a fairy tale, while men see it as a woman doing something enjoyable with them, like going to a movie, restaurant, or sporting event together.

Lovers who practice sacred sexuality often begin their sex session with a dedication to each other and their practice, such as the following:

→ I respect you.
→ You are an important part of my universe.
→ I honor the love we share.
→ I wish for our love to keep us connected to each other and the universe.
→ I cherish you.
→ You bring joy to my spirit.
→ I want you in my life forever.
→ Enter my heart.
→ Look into my eyes.
→ I want to share my life with you.
→ Take my hand.

Any well-written book on Tantric sex or the Kama Sutra should offer suggestions for what you and your lover can say. Or for a more far-reaching experience, you and your partner could enroll in a Tantric workshop and discover your most profound, ecstatic lovers within.

I-WANT-TO-GET-IN-YOUR-PANTS INSPIRATION

And there lay the lovers, lip-locked
Delirious, infinitely thirsting
Each wanting to go completely
inside the other

Now read the text again slowly, allowing yourself to visualize the scene. What are you feeling? These lines by the sixth century Roman poet Paulus Silentiarius are a fine example of how words can be at once sensual and seductive. Eros-driven writings like these will likely have you fanning yourself—if not a whole lot more. The objective is to fan the flames of desire. To help you achieve this objective, there are a number of resources you can turn to, starting with erotic books and poetry, which are usually shelved in separate sections in most bookstores. You can also listen to erotic stories on audiotape or CD, or watch a sexy film you find at a video store (films with R or X ratings are usually not considered all-out porn). Investing some time and researching your erotic talk material is sure to pay off, as Shea knows: "My partners have tended to say they like that I'm well-read or have a certain sense of humor, so that's the verbal stuff I've concentrated on."

And there lay the lovers,
lip-locked
Delirious, infinitely thirsting
Each wanting to go completely
inside the other

Here's your first reading assignment:
"She Performed as Never Before,"
written in the twelfth century by Javadeva.

She performed as never before throughout the course
Of the conflict of love, to win, lying over his beautiful
Body, to triumph over her lover;
And so through taking the active part her thighs grew
Lifeless, and languid her vine-like arms, and her
Heart beat fast, and her eyes grew heavy and closed;
For how many women prevail in the male performance!

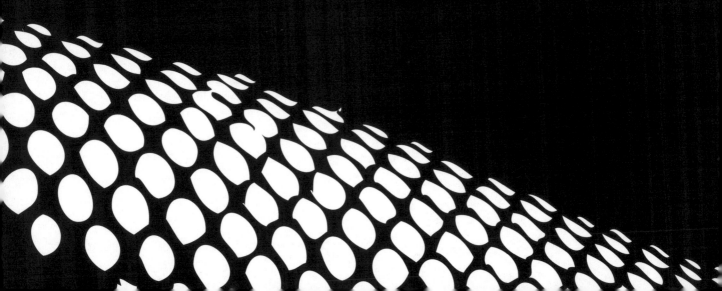

In the morning most wondrous, the heart of her lord
Was smitten with arrows of Love, arrows which went
Through his eyes,

Arrows which were her nail-scratched bosom, her reddened
Sleep-denied eyes, her crimson lips from a bath
Of kisses, her hair disarranged with the flowers awry,
And her girdle all loose and slipping.

With hair knot loosened and stray locks waving, her
Cheeks perspiring, her glitter of bimba lips impaired,
And the necklace of pearls not appearing fair because
Of her jar-shaped breasts being denuded,
And her belt, her glittering girdle, dimmed in beauty,
And all of a sudden placing her hands on her naked
Breasts, and over her naked loins, to hide them, and
Looking embarrassed;
Even so, with her tender loveliness ravaged,
She continued to please!

No one is expecting you to be quite this elaborate in your efforts. If your words are chosen carefully and expressed with ardor, even a little says a lot—for example, "Just let me watch you."

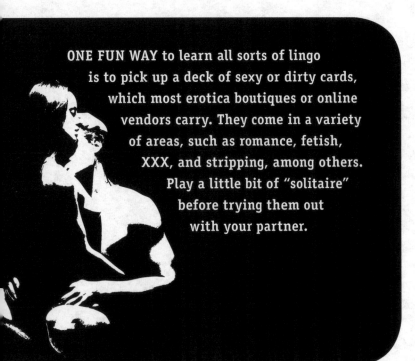

ONE FUN WAY to learn all sorts of lingo is to pick up a deck of sexy or dirty cards, which most erotica boutiques or online vendors carry. They come in a variety of areas, such as romance, fetish, XXX, and stripping, among others. Play a little bit of "solitaire" before trying them out with your partner.

GETTING DOWN 'N DIRTY INSPIRATION

"Dirty. Dirty, dirty, dirty. Slimy, nasty, crude, vile. I like all of the words that you're not supposed to say with the lights on, especially in mixed company." Like Lou, some people just like their sex talk dirty.

Porn is an obvious source for dirty-talk inspiration, but many people feel they have better results when they reach for hardcore literature, such as *Penthouse Forum*, that tends to be less cheesy. Here's a snippet:

"My chin was dripping with Jill-juice as she pulled my mouth up to hers. Her tongue probed my mouth, as if I were hiding something from her. As I lowered my head to her tits, Jill said, 'I love the taste of my pussy. Kiss me again.' I pressed my mouth against hers and ran my tongue all over her face."

As you pour over the lit that you've discovered online or in your bookstore's adult/romantic fiction, poetry anthologies, or gay and lesbian sections, you'll start to pick up on recurring themes and elements that can guide you in composing your own written or aural efforts. Here are some tips. You'll want to . . .

Make it wet. Slick, dripping, juicy, slippery, gushing, seeping, slithery . . . People give the impression that they're squeamish about bodily fluids, but when it comes to getting down and dirty, they're all about sexual hydraulics: "Now take off those soaking wet tights and rub your clit against mine."

Keep it action-oriented. Ram, hump, thrust, stick, pull, push, grab, touch, fondle, rub, screw, play, tease, squeeze, pump, grind, brush, jam, spank: "Finger-fuck me while he watches."

Use your mouth. Lick, eat, swallow, drink, kiss, chew, nibble, suck, bite, blow: "I'm going to lick you clean."

Stimulate the senses. Have fun tapping them all, though smell and taste get the most play: "Sit on my face. I'm going to eat you till you can't stay upright any more."

Be descriptive. Here are some great words to use: throbbing, warm, aching, erect, hungry, tight, big, stiff, huge, strong, swollen, soft, nasty, hard, firm, luscious, naked, massive, steamy, heaving, hung, well-hung, insatiable.

If print and film aren't enough inspiration to enliven your dirty talk, calling a sex line can give you plenty of ideas. To find the phone numbers for these pay-per-minute calls, check online or in the back pages of your city paper.

Dear Dirty Diary

Consider maintaining an erotic diary. It could include anything that strikes your fancy and might serve as inspiration—from keeping track of sex dreams to honest reactions to sexual liaisons about what worked and what didn't. You can also use this book of private thoughts to jot down words, lines of verse, phrases, quotes, short stories . . . whatever juicy material you discover that lights your fuse or gives you revelations that you'd like to recall and act on later. Think of it as your secret stash of language and insights that propel you toward pleasure.

Sound: The Ultimate Aphrodisiac

An aphrodisiac is anything that excites. And when it comes to awakening and boosting your sexual desire, nothing is so readily at your disposal—or quite as effective—as the amorous, indecent, or soulful sounds that emanate from your mouth. Sexy talk is an enchanting way to seduce your lover and to stay bewitched. Most people love the ego boost of hearing "I want you," and they thrill to the adulation and affirmation that comes from knowing that their partner is sexually satisfied. Charlotte agrees wholeheartedly: "You want to feel like you're the best lover they have ever had, and making noise or sexy talk does just that."

Eroticizing each other with talk has major payoffs. Erotic talk teases your brain, setting it ablaze and boosting the mind-body connection that's needed for the best sex. From natural sounds to talking dirty, aural sex bolsters your sexual response cycle. In fueling your sexual desire and excitement, your body sends more blood to the genitals, making you even more sensitive to stimulation. It also amps up your lover's enthusiasm, as Michael can affirm: "Any kind of aural positive reinforcement is great. It lets me know what I am doing is good. So I'll do it more." In a nutshell, aural efforts make for a more intense, more erotic, hotter experience.

From Panting to Putting It Out There: Finding Your Voice

Before we jump into our first "voice lesson," let's deal with a fundamental issue. When you work your magic, we don't want anything vexing you. From our earliest years, we are told to be quiet and speak only when spoken to; nobody wants a peep out of us unless we've got something important to say, have an urgent question, or are cheering on a sports team. Screaming, crying, shouting, laughing out loud, pleading, whining—these are all discouraged, for the most part.

But the truth is, we need to voice our emotions and it's okay to challenge some of the absurd taboos that surround making noise—all kinds of noise. And it's okay to be loud about it.

This includes your sex life. When it comes to sexual expression, making your innermost longings, feelings, and needs known is a good and healthy practice. Sound effects, whether they be grunting, moaning, shrieking, purring, or giggling, are all wonderful because they:

→ Indicate that you're becoming incredibly aroused
→ Signify that you're having a fantastic time
→ Serve as a declaration of your affection and passion
→ Affirm a job well done
→ State what you need and how

So dare yourself to be eloquent, graphic, teasing, or naughty. Dig down deep, tap into your sensuous nature, and know no fear in unfurling your passion. Take risks in describing what you want, articulating your needs, and declaring how your intimate experiences affect you. This may seem like a tall order now, but you *can* do it—just promise yourself that you won't let anything hold you back.

A Word with the Men

Most resources about the role of sound with sex or erotic talk tend to focus on women. Sex therapists, educators, and writers are always encouraging them to be vocal when getting down and dirty—and rightfully so. Traditionally, women have been expected to stifle their sexuality, to stay silent. But what about men? It's either assumed that they have no sex communication issues or that it's perfectly acceptable for them to be mute. Nothing could be farther from the truth.

While it's fine to be stereotypically "manly" and unemotional in your day-to-day affairs, sex is not a time for keeping up appearances. It is not the time to be distant or stoic. Unless it's a phallus, nobody wants a stiff in bed. Aziza certainly doesn't, and she makes sure that her lovers are nothing less than her erotic talk equals: "I feel that it's very important to have the freedom to be vocal in bed. My ex was always quiet and I was very insecure about that. I felt he wasn't enjoying me or that he was withholding the pleasure of knowing I pleased him from me. That was not good. The partners I choose now tend to be sexually secure men and their vocal expressions and sexy talk always impacts sex for the better!"

BRAIN RESEARCH on male-female communication styles helps to explain a lot of the general communication that takes place in a relationship. In using the left-brain side of their brain more than both sides, as women do, males tend to prefer more direct communication. They like to be coached. This is easy, if you're a lover who likes to take charge!

They say you never forget your first time, and for me the ones having to do with sound in many ways stand out best. I'll never forget the first time I could actually hear what a (now ex) lover was experiencing. He let out a moan, then another one—then a cry, and then another one, as he pulled me up to hold me as he erupted into orgasm. His body writhing against mine, his damp forehead resting on mine, his sweet breath pulsing "ooh's" onto my face. . . . I felt awestruck by what I was witnessing, and especially by what I was hearing. It was beautiful. It was the first time a lover had truly let himself go in conveying his pleasure with vocal applause.

So don't let being a guy—or playing up to the stereotypes—trump your game in the sack. Making noise is a sign that you're secure with yourself, that you're confident in your sexuality, and that you're unafraid to embrace and share your sexual response. Those are the qualities that make for a real man in bed, and they are supersexy to your lover. Like you, your partner wants to know that you're having the time of your life. Whether you're grunting, moaning, or howling, you're letting your partner know that you are in the moment and that you couldn't be any happier.

Loading Up Your Auditory Ammo

Now that you have a better sense of the incredible impact sound can have on our mind, body, and spirit, you may be thinking, *If sound has that much influence on me and my partner, what in the world should come out of my mouth?* It's important to realize that *what* you say is not nearly as important as the way you say it.

Consider Hollywood icon Marilyn Monroe's classic delivery of "Happy Birthday" to President John F. Kennedy back in 1962. Sinfully sweet and scorching hot, Monroe gave one of her most memorable performances, turning a wholesome song into what's known on the street these days as a type of "eargasm" (the sensation one gets listening to a dramatic musical climax).

Erotic Talk Action Plan: Discovering Your Sexual Core

As Marilyn Monroe illustrated so well, when it comes to making an aural impression, your aim is to have an aesthetically pleasing voice. In erotic talk, this means sounding warm, rhythmic, rich, and soothing. You want your lustful lingo to practically drip from your lips. You want your wanton whispers to infiltrate your lover's core, causing ripples of insatiable desire.

Even if you consider yourself a natural born crooner, it never hurts to tune your instrument for delivering an arresting eargasm. The following exercises are all geared toward optimizing the quality of your oral sound production:

1. Warming up your vocal chords
2. Expanding your waistline
3. Letting go
4. Developing a sexier breath
5. Recording your orgasm
6. Self-pleasuring

Whether you choose to do these in a single sitting or slowly over time, these exercises will help you get in touch with your sensual energy, stir up with your vocal abilities, become more erotic, and take command of your sound. As you learn to tap your vocal vibrations in a way that makes your lover's nether regions tingle, your voice will become an aural art form that transforms you into a sexy sorcerer. Transfixed, your lover will become putty in your hands. Sexing up your sound is the ultimate erotic elixir, from setting the mood to kicking things up a notch to pushing your partner over the edge into ecstasy. It's your sure-fire tactic that guarantees sizzling sex.

Note: To resolve feelings of discomfort or embarrassment, and to create an atmosphere of safety and relaxation in which to launch your efforts, make sure to set aside adequate private time.

To get you on your vocal erotic talk way, we're going to stimulate the energy in your body using the storehouse of it situated in your throat. Known as the fifth chakra, this energy center is in charge of your creative expression, action, will, choices, telepathy, and spoken word. It controls your ability to communicate, and when balanced, you can speak your dreams and ask for your wants, helping some to come true. Getting in tune with this energy center is getting in touch with your spirit and your sexual spirituality in a whole new way.

Before doing the following meditation, size up the health of this energy center, since doing so helps gauge the ease with which you express yourself:

➔ Do you take responsibility for your own needs?
➔ Do you surrender your personal will to truthfulness (versus deceit)?
➔ Are you able to express your personality and creativity relatively easily?
➔ Are you open and honest with yourself and others?

TIME: 30 minutes

LUST-INDUCING LOCATION: a place at home like a den or sun room, where you practice yoga or meditation (or would if you did)

MATERIALS: a cup of salt water

PEAKING POTENTIAL: 2+—you're charging yourself with your life force!

The following are physical signs and symptoms indicating that you should attend to the health of your vocal energy center:

Sore throat

Mouth ulcers

Scoliosis

Swollen glands

Thyroid dysfunctions

Laryngitis

Strep throat

Speech impediment

Gum or tooth problems

Addiction

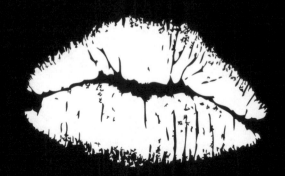

The energy center based in your throat governs the thyroid, trachea, mouth, neck vertebrae, teeth, gums, esophagus, parathyroid, and hypothalamus. Difficulty releasing your truths, attitudes, anger, and displeasure can harm your body and spirit because unexpressed emotions constrict this energy center.

To express yourself to the fullest during erotic talk practices—and to stimulate your body's energy—perform the following ritual at least a couple of times per week (daily practice is ideal for anyone with related health issues):

1. Gargle with room-temperature salt water and spit it out. Then make yourself comfortable in a seated, cross-legged position on the floor.
2. Close your eyes and focus on the color turquoise or Russian blue (this is the color that represents your throat center).
3. Note how you're feeling and the quality of your thoughts. Are they calm? Full of a certain emotion? Bringing up a particular memory?
4. Pay attention to any sensations in your body.
5. Take slow, deep breaths, visualizing that you're warming your throat as you channel your breath to your core, and release any tensions. Release any noises that arise in your throat.
6. Close this exercise by completing the following affirmations:
   - I express my sexual creativity by . . .
   - I express myself easily and joyfully with a partner by . . .
   - When it comes to my sensuality, I want to . . .
   - I hope for . . . /dream of . . . , and I follow through with heart.

Who says that a bigger waistline can't make for better sex? When it comes to your sound potential, it most certainly does. You need to breathe through your diaphragm to achieve richer, fuller, sexier sounds. Plus, being in control of your diaphragm extends your voice

range. Normal breathing tends to be shallow and uses only the top half of your lungs, whereas expanding your diaphragm uses the whole lung. This action is particularly effective in producing husky, throaty, breathy—terribly erotic—sounds.

To tune into and tune up your vocal energy, you're going to practice breathing from your diaphragm. Be sure to do the following in a warm, comfortable space:

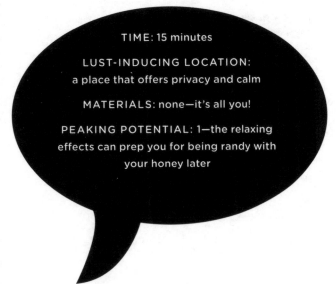

TIME: 15 minutes

LUST-INDUCING LOCATION:
a place that offers privacy and calm

MATERIALS: none—it's all you!

PEAKING POTENTIAL: 1—the relaxing effects can prep you for being randy with your honey later

1. Identify your diaphragm, the area between your chest and abdomen just above your waist. You can do this by lying on your back, placing the palm of your hand on this area, and inhaling deeply through your nose. Your midsection should push your hand up as it expands, with your chest and shoulders staying relaxed. This is where you want your breath to come from when it's time to talk sexy.

2. Take a deep breath, and as you slowly exhale, say "Ahhh . . ." until you run out of air. Repeat several times.

3. In seeking to further improve your exhalation, inhale, purse your lips, and draw your abs in gently as you exhale to free your diaphragm. Repeat for several breaths.

4. Once you're comfortable with step 3, pause several times as you breathe in, using a yoga breath control technique known as "viloma pranayama." (*Viloma* means "to go against natural order.")

5. Pause several times as you exhale in further practicing this breath.

Make a point of practicing this exercise regularly. It will expand your breathing and make you more relaxed for your erotic talk efforts and life events in general. Delivering increased energy and relaxation, this practice puts you in the optimal state for seeing your lover because it makes you more receptive to and in the mood for sex.

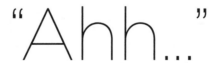

"Ahh..."

Building on the diaphragm control you mastered in the previous exercise, now you're going to practice different sounds that lovers frequently make in the bedroom. As you make the following sounds, connect with the emotions that arise. Allow yourself to get louder and louder with each expression. Give yourself permission to let go. You'll see your practice starts with allowing yourself to say "Yes!"—one of the sexiest words around. Whenever you find yourself struggling to let loose during any of the following steps, return to building up your "Yes!" response, and then revisit the sound that made you struggle with renewed aural energy.

TIME: 15 minutes

LUST-INDUCING LOCATION:
after scheduling private time, slip into your bedroom, bathroom, or for the terribly shy, a good-size closet

MATERIALS: if playing music puts you at ease, have your stereo, MP3 player, or laptop handy

PEAKING POTENTIAL: 2—releasing sound waves fueled with feeling has the potential to trigger an emotional orgasm (or orgasm of the heart), an experience familiar to Tantric sex practitioners; for women, imagining sexual fantasies while making erotic sounds and channeling their breath to their pelvic core can also lead to an extragenital orgasm (climax without genital stimulation), so get ready to focus on making some noise—and enjoying your body's spontaneous, climactic responses!

1. Start saying "Yes," and gradually get louder and louder and say it with more conviction. Whether you're a man or woman, draw inspiration from the infamous scene from *When Harry Met Sally* when Meg Ryan mimics having an orgasm. (For a refresher, you can check out Meg's scene online at YouTube.)

2. Let your loud "Yes!"s turn to deep breathing and loud sighs.

3. As you come down, tune into your voice by humming to relax.

4. Let out little moans, much like the sound you'd make when you see an adorable puppy.

5. As you get more accustomed to hearing yourself, make the following sounds. If it helps, imagine an animal that makes a similar sound, or pretend that you're at a yoga class where students are given permission to get a little zany, let down their guard, and tap into their animalistic or primitive sides:

- Whimper (like an adoring dog eager to see its owner)
- Cry (like loved ones being reunited)
- Shriek (like a bird of prey going in for the kill)
- Howl (like a wolf calling its mate)
- Grunt (like a pig eager for its feast)
- Growl (like a lion fiercely protecting its lair)
- Laugh (like a hyena devouring a meal)
- Pant (like an Olympic athlete having just crossed the finish line)
- Purr (like a cat in heat)
- Giggle (like a happy baby)

6. As you make each of these noises, tune into any physical stirrings they provoke.

7. Consider which of those sounds might be a turn-on in bed!

This type of breath work will energize and relax you during erotic talk, plus it will make you more alluring as you learn the power of effective pauses that can be good for teasing and titillating.

TIME: 15+ minutes

LUST-INDUCING LOCATION: any place you can sound sexy without restraint or risk of shutting down your sexual response (e.g., where you needn't worry that anyone might hear you)

MATERIALS: music, if desired

PEAKING POTENTIAL: 2—higher if you get carried away with yourself!

1. Sit in a meditative, cross-legged position and relax.
2. Take a deep breath in, and, on the exhale, let it go naturally.
3. As you inhale, pretend that you're sipping the breath through a straw and gently constrict the opening of your throat so that it creates resistance against the incoming air. Stay relaxed.
4. As you exhale, gently push the breath out against the resistance, making sure that your exhalation is not shorter than your inhalation.
5. As you get the hang of this breath, eventually inhale and focus on creating a soothing, pleasing sound that isn't hurried or forced. You're aiming for a long, smooth breath.
6. With practice, as you feel more in command of this type of breathing, make sexy sounds like, "Ooo," "Ohh," "Mmm," and "Aww" with each exhale.

7. Eventually, work yourself to a point where you can "think off." Here, you think yourself to orgasm by giving yourself over to the naughty thoughts in your head. Staying in control of your breath, allow yourself to react to sexual scenarios that cause your heart to skip a beat. This could involve remembering the first time you had sex with your partner, getting a loving massage, being serviced by two total knockouts at the same time, having a quickie on a quiet night train, being penetrated while performing oral sex on someone else. . . . Everyone is going to have their own forte, so go with what works for you, noticing your breath as your mind's movie reel shifts into high gear.

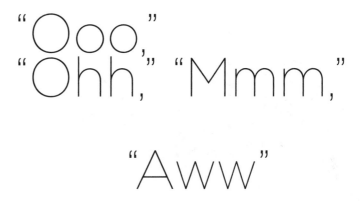

"Ooo," "Ohh," "Mmm," "Aww"

To record your climax for your lover:

1. Arrange your self-pleasuring scene.
2. Plug in your computer microphone. (Note: A hands-free headset is terrific because it allows you to put the mic right up against your lips.)

3. Do a test run, starting with the mic. Hit "record," and do what it takes to bring on a heart-stopping orgasmic reaction, keeping it to no more than a couple of minutes. Hit "stop," and then listen to the results. (For those of you using a phone, leave yourself a voicemail. You can then go to a service like GotVoice.com to set up an account for downloading your voicemail messages from your phone to your computer.)
4. Continue until you're satisfied (pleased *and* sexually gratified) with the recording.
5. Save your file in a safe place.
6. When you're ready to send it, go to the File menu in Audacity and click "Export Selection to MP3."
7. At the prompt, enter your file name.
8. Now send the MP3 file to your lucky lover by attaching it to an e-mail like you would any other file.

TIME: 30 minutes, but only if you're a perfectionist or you listen to your recording obsessively before you send this "O"

LUST-INDUCING LOCATION: at your computer

MATERIALS: Audacity, a free audio editing application available at audacity.sourceforge.net, or an MP3 player with a microphone attachment, a cell phone or a PDA with a "voice memo" feature, plus the ability to create MP3s, the digital audio recording format, on your computer

PEAKING POTENTIAL: 2.5—hearing yourself come can make your body want to feel your orgasm for real

Sex educators and therapists frequently advise people to masturbate if they want to have better sex. That's because you need to find out what works for you on your own before sharing the information with a partner. The same goes for erotic talk. You've been presented with various examples of heart-thumping erotic talk to see which can transport you to a transcendent sex state. Now it's time to test out the material—on yourself. This kind of solo rehearsal allows you to deal with your inhibitions and desensitize yourself to certain words or phrases while you connect with your wants, needs, and sexual energy.

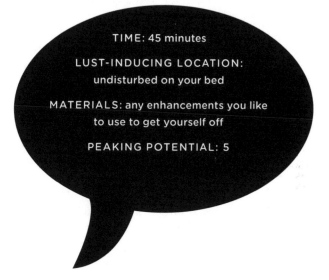

TIME: 45 minutes

LUST-INDUCING LOCATION:
undisturbed on your bed

MATERIALS: any enhancements you like
to use to get yourself off

PEAKING POTENTIAL: 5

This exercise is set up so that you'll probably want to pleasure yourself on more than one occasion (which makes for only more good times to be had). Just how often you get off comes down to how thoroughly you're able to lose yourself in the fantasy each erotic theme triggers and ride it for what it's worth.

There are two ways to go about this exercise: You can get yourself in the mood by masturbating before reading a scenario, or wait and see if you have a libidinal reaction to what you read.

1. Carefully read and think about each scenario in the "Erotic Talk Triggers" section on page 88, letting yourself feel your reactions to an attractive someone saying each statement to you or vice versa.

2. Consider what it is about this type of erotic talk that might turn you on, noting your reactions, if any, and then running with it. (Note: Pay attention to whether the comment turns you on or off or whether it's no-go territory given your current relationship, because this can make a huge difference in what feels good.)

3. Play with yourself as you build the plot in your head. At first, you may only be able to breathe or moan in response to your thoughts.

4. Eventually, think out loud as though your lover were there with you, saying your sexy thoughts as they come to you. Start by saying your lover's name, as though you could never tire of hearing it.

5. Begin to utter sexy words or phrases to your fantasy lover(s). Don't censor your thoughts! You can say anything you want. Just don't forget your natural sounds.

6. Don't worry about your delivery or how you sound. You just want to go with what's natural, getting your sexy talk out there. If it doesn't feel good to hear it, who cares? You're alone, right? You have the ability to create and influence the kind of erotic talk experience you're after. Allow yourself to feel the fear and do it anyway.

7. Really increase talking to yourself as you approach orgasm for greater intensity. In many cases, this will bring your orgasm on faster.

8. Consider going back to the themes or reactions that worked well for you. What tones might make your efforts easier or sexier? Sex kitten-like, dominating, or breathier? We're not interested in practice making perfect here; instead, you're rehearsing to build your comfort level. Dealing with all of your performance jitters here will put you at ease when it really matters.

Erotic Talk Triggers

Expressing a need for another: "I need you in the worst way!"

Being confessional while feeling sexually piqued in a public place: "I'm not wearing any panties," or "Wouldn't you know? I'm going commando."

Being seductive while being videotaped: "Do I make you think nasty thoughts?"

Making a request about this masturbation session: "Please let me watch."

Taking a lover's breath away after learning you're crazy about each other:

"How can I not think of you?"

Hearing someone desire you during a strip tease: "You make me *so* hard."

Telling someone you desire him or her: "I want to feel your body writhing with pleasure as I . . . "

Stating a devotion prior to a Tantric sex session: "I worship the love inside you."

Being dominant during an orgy: "Put your face between my thighs, and your ass in the air!"

Being dominated during a bondage session: "Do you want me to tie you down?"

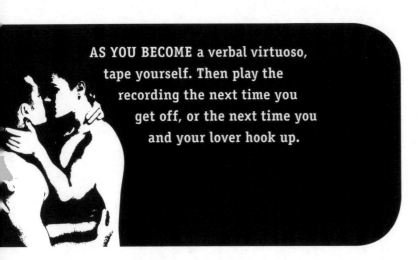

AS YOU BECOME a verbal virtuoso, tape yourself. Then play the recording the next time you get off, or the next time you and your lover hook up.

Chapter 2 Check-In

Chapter 2 sought to examine your mind-set about erotic talk. In evaluating your performance, answer the following:

→ Do you have an open-minded, healthy attitude that will bring you all that erotic talk has to offer? Or do you feel that you're your own worst enemy in this effort when it comes to verbal performance anxiety?

→ Which sources of inspiration for erotic talk would you like to further explore? When and how are you going to make that happen?

→ Do you need to give yourself a pep talk or confidence booster when it comes to certain types of sexy talk?

→ Were the throat center chakra and breath work valuable? Why or why not? How can your reactions to those exercises be helping or hurting your efforts?

This chapter sought to motivate you in your ability to make all types of noise for your eventual sexual enjoyment. In processing what the experience was like for you, gauge how well you think you did in terms of:

→ Finding your voice. Was it a challenge? Do you feel that you need more work? If so, what might have held you back from reaching the more aphrodisiac-type sounds you hope to one day let loose? Or are you at a much better starting point than you realized?

→ Tuning into your sensations simply by getting vocal. Which ones roused emotions? Which have the potential to become more sensual or sexual?

→ In considering the self-pleasuring sessions, which sexy talk situations were amazing, so-so, or not worth trying with somebody?

→ What was it like to masturbate while making sounds? What were your thoughts, emotions, and sensations?

→ What do you need from your partner to make this kind of erotic talk happen?

Make a pledge to maintain your efforts—to strengthen and expand your diaphragm, to stimulate your vocal energy center, and to fire up and free your most primal, sensual sounds. Revisit these exercises often—and invite your lover to join in for what can be a surprising, revealing, and playful bonding experience as you both master the art of erotic talk.

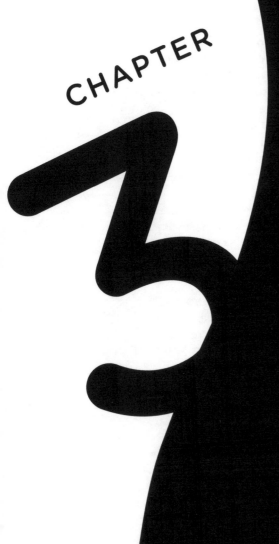

Practice Makes Perfect: Using Erotic Talk to Get the Sex You Want

IN CHAPTER 3, YOU'LL LEARN HOW TO:

☞ Master the rules of erotic engagement.

☞ Share each other's deepest sexual thoughts.

☞ Provide your partner with positive feedback and support.

☞ Work toward sexual compatibility.

☞ Invite your lover to a steamy show and tell.

☞ Give a whole new slip of the tongue.

☞ Test your dirty talk talents

Here you are, ready to

captivate your lover with stimulating thrills and heartfelt provocation with no more than what is on the tip of your tongue. It's time to tap your sexual sensibilities and have the aural sex many only dream of having. In this chapter, we'll cover hot topics that boost sexual relationships, and you'll see what needs to be done when you and your lover aren't on the same page sexually speaking. You'll learn about your bodies and sexual response in a whole new way. And finally, you'll introduce all of the erotic talk you want in the sack to bring a sizzle to your sexcapades.

IN LAUNCHING SEX TALK ATTEMPTS, the one thing you don't want to do is to put your lover on the spot: "Honey, I'm home! Let's talk about sex, okay?" Some people can communicate about sex easily and on the fly, while others believe that there is a time and place to talk about sex.

Because topics related to sex are highly personal and revealing, lovers can be a bit thrown off if they're not given a head's up. Even when done with the best of intentions, springing a sex talk on someone can actually cause them to withdraw more than come out of their shell.

I am reminded of a sweet and caring lover, unsure if he was pleasing me, who asked me what I liked in bed. Since we hadn't been sleeping together for long, and since I was being patient and comfortable with the fact that we were slowly connecting, I was thrown off. I hadn't yet considered what I would like to do differently with him because I was still trying to absorb the newness of us. I felt totally put on the spot and didn't know what to say. The pressure of my work as a sex expert didn't make it easier. Shouldn't I have a file in my head of what I love, what I don't like, what I hope to try, what I need to fine-tune . . . no matter with whom? I shut down and became defensive, responding with sarcasm, "Why don't you read one of my books?" Not my finest moment.

To avoid missteps, you should let your lover know that you'd like to arrange a relaxed, agreeable time to talk about sex. Reassure your lover that the goal of conversations like these is to share positive points of your relationship, discuss ideas for getting more connected, and assess your physical and emotional needs when it comes to being intimate.

Make a date to talk. Then share the questions and topics in this chapter for review ahead of time so that both of you feel prepared.

RULES OF ENGAGEMENT

Before embarking on your sex talk "date," settle on your rules of engagement, using the following as jumping-off points:

➜ Give yourselves permission to have this date without any interruptions or distractions, to be open, and to talk about sex.

➜ State your needs, wants, and limits.

➜ Be sincere and genuine, because this contributes to each person's sense of safety, respect, and feeling valued.

➜ Respect and support your partner in the process.

➜ Stay positive and use constructive language (in other words, don't criticize).

➜ Ask for a "time-out" if necessary (e.g., to gather your thoughts if something that comes up takes you by surprise).

➜ Give each other your undivided attention.

➜ Be aware of what you're thinking and how that makes you feel.

➜ Be mindful of what you say and how you say it.

➜ Make it okay to stumble, laugh, blush.

Whether you've known your lover for one month or one decade, you stand to gain a deeper understanding from this kind of exchange. You want to learn everything you can about this one very special human being's sexuality and how it's experienced and expressed. In developing your true intimacy and talking about your sex life, you will slowly unearth your lover's personal identity as a sexual human being. That process can be extremely erotic in and of itself.

The Importance of Nonverbals

While this book is overwhelmingly about what comes out of your mouth, we shouldn't overlook the nonverbal messages you send your lover when you communicate about sex. (Nonverbals make up 93 percent of the in-person communication we experience.) Pay attention to body language when you're having a sex talk.

Remember the following tips:

➜ Don't underestimate the power of eye contact. Your lover will feel more enchanted and connected to you if you hold each other's gaze. Moreover, research has found that maintaining eye contact boosts one's attractiveness.

➜ Be open and receptive in your body language. Lean forward and try not to cross your arms or legs.

➜ Keep your face animated. Research shows that looking alert and engaged makes you more attractive than keeping an expressionless face.

➜ Don't angle your body away from your partner, as this is can be interpreted as losing interest in or emotionally turning away from your lover.

➜ Don't lean backward or support your head with one hand, since this can indicate boredom.

➜ Don't fake a smile. People can tell instantly when your expression isn't genuine.

GETTING YOUR COMMUNICATION styles in sync is in your better interest. Similarities in a couple's social and communication skills are important predictors of attraction and marital satisfaction. Both of these vital relationship components promote attraction by fostering enjoyable interactions.

For date night, you and your partner will complete a series of sentences or answer questions that are designed to reveal more about each other's sexual thoughts. Beforehand, take the time to individually read through the statements and questions, deciding which you'd like to address and considering your responses. Then, during your date, you can pose one of the questions to your partner or offer your completion of a sentence about sex.

To begin, remind each other about the ground rules you established in chapter 1 and recognize what's expected from both of you in sharing and providing erotic feedback.

Here are some tips for sharing:

→ Be specific. Effective communication is in the details.
→ Be open to receiving feedback.
→ Ask questions that are open-ended. Questions requiring no more than a yes or no response limit the amount of information you will get from your partner.

→ Listen carefully and ask for clarification if necessary: "Did I understand you fully?" "Am I hearing you clearly?" "What else is there for you?" "Is there anything I'm missing?"
→ Invite fuller responses by saying, "I'm listening" or "Tell me more."
→ Give honest and caring feedback.

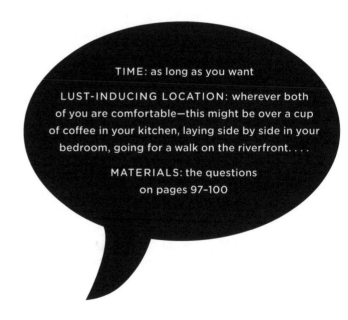

TIME: as long as you want

LUST-INDUCING LOCATION: wherever both of you are comfortable—this might be over a cup of coffee in your kitchen, laying side by side in your bedroom, going for a walk on the riverfront. . . .

MATERIALS: the questions on pages 97–100

Concentrate on what your partner is saying; don't get distracted by what your response will be. In other words, be present.

Validate your partner's feelings by acknowledging his or her perspectives: "I didn't know that you felt that way. Let's talk about what I/we can do."

Know that it's okay to feel unsure or to need more time to reflect: "Can I get back to you? I need to think about that."

Follow up later or the next day with words that reinforce the importance of what you've shared: "I'm glad we talked."

And here are some tips on what not to do:

→ Don't change the subject.
→ Don't minimize or dismiss your partner's fears, worries, or dreams.
→ Don't be a know-it-all.
→ Don't interrupt or finish your partner's sentences.

→ Avoid using "always" or "never"—doing so makes you come across as defensive and adversarial.
→ Avoid "should" statements.
→ Don't speak in a domineering, hostile, or sarcastic tone.

I know, you're eager to dive in, but one more important bit of advice: Don't exhaust your lover when it comes to erotic talk expectations. Yes, it's exciting, and yes, it can be easy to lose yourselves in a number of ways. But people can feel fatigued from the intensity of the sharing that takes place, especially if they're digging up old hurts or negative past experiences. Take a break from discussing your sex life when this happens, even if it's for days or weeks.

Ready? Start by completing the sentences on the next page, honing in on the ones you feel apply to your current sexual needs. Then look over the list of topics that follow the Sex Sentence Completion exercise to see if they spark further discussion.

Note: Do not feel obligated to address all of these topics, especially in one sitting. Just take your time to thoughtfully consider each.

Sex Sentence Completion

→ What I like about our sex life is that . . .
→ What it comes to intense orgasms, I . . .
→ Something I don't care for is . . .
→ Something I'm really curious about is . . .
→ I've always wanted to try . . .
→ One thing I'd like from you . . .
→ One thing that worries me . . .
→ I really like it when you . . .
→ My expectations around sex involve . . .
→ Reasons I like to have sex are . . .
→ To me, sex is about . . .
→ For me, I would like for the sex we have to be about . . .

Sex Trivia

→ How much sex do you want? How much sex is realistic?
→ Have you noticed that your sex drive is higher during a certain time of day (e.g., morning, afternoon, evening)?
→ Does your sex drive vary throughout the month? If so, when?
→ (For women) My monthly menstrual cycle affects my sexual desire in that. . . .
→ Over time, I feel like my sex drive and sexual performance have . . .
→ How do you initiate sex? Would you prefer that one person do so more than the other? If so, why?
→ Do you feel obligated to have sex if you're the one not in the mood? How do you feel when you give in to requests or pressures to put out?
→ When it comes to sexual spontaneity, I . . .
→ When it comes to prearranged sexual encounters, like Sunday morning sex, I . . .

Sexual Health

→ Is it in our best interest to use contraceptives? Does using them or not using them impact our sexual intimacy for better or for worse?

→ Are we satisfied and comfortable with the type of birth control that we're using?

→ Should we be protecting ourselves from sexually transmitted infections by using condoms or dental dams?

→ Are we satisfied with our safer sex practices?

→ Do we have a back-up plan if the contraceptives aren't used correctly or consistently? If not, what should it be?

→ Have we both been tested for sexually transmitted infections, including HIV? If not, is there a need? If there is, how should we go about doing this?

Sexual Dynamics

→ What are your thoughts around lovers being aggressive versus passive?

→ When it comes to giving and receiving sexual pleasure, I prefer that . . .

→ When I get turned down for sex, I . . .

→ Sometimes I feel obligated to . . .

→ When my partner is unwilling to do a particular sex act, I . . .

→ When I'm unwilling to do something my partner asks for, I . . .

→ Is sex ever used as a bargaining tool? Do either of you withhold sex as punishment? How does this make you feel?

→ For me, sexual variety is . . .

→ I see sex versus making love as . . .

→ Emotions that enhance our sex life for the better include . . .

→ Emotions that contaminate our sex life are . . .

→ Religious beliefs playing into my ability to be sexual are . . .

- → I deal with sexual disappointment by . . .
- → I react to my sexual desires by . . .
- → I feel that you react to my sexual desires by . . .

Sexual Preferences

- → Foreplay, for me, is ideal when it involves . . . (e.g., lights, clothing, places)
- → Types of foreplay I don't care for include . . .
- → During foreplay, for me to eventually reach peak sexual responsiveness, I need . . .
- → Affectionate touches I like are . . .
- → How much kissing do you like? How important is making out as a form of foreplay? Do you like kissing to continue throughout sexual intercourse?
- → My most favorite positions include . . .
- → My least favorite positions include . . .
- → During oral sex, I like . . .
- → Sex acts that really turn me on are . . .
- → Sex acts that are a turn-off are . . .
- → My reactions to sacred sex are that it . . .
- → Kinky sexual behaviors I'm open to include . . .
- → Kinky sexual behaviors I have trouble getting into include . . .
- → I fantasize about experimenting with . . .
- → My feelings around masturbation are that . . .
- → When it comes to mutual masturbation . . .
- → My feelings around cuddling are that . . .
- → After making love, I . . .
- → I'm curious about having sex in/on/at . . .

Sexual Response

→ When it comes to sexual satisfaction, I am all about . . .

→ Do we pay attention to each other's sexual needs?

→ Is the level of satisfaction in our sex life equal? Does it need to be?

→ When it comes to being orgasmic, I weigh this reaction as being . . .

→ When it comes to my sex drive, it has been . . .

→ When it comes to my ability to be sexually intimate, I . . .

→ My perception of myself (weight, appearance, etc.) affects my sex life in that . . .

→ How intimate do I feel during sex?

After each sex talk, process what the experience was like for you. Answering these questions can be very difficult: You may not like everything you hear, and you might even question your sexual compatibility as a couple (if this is the case, see the next section, "Sexual Compatibility"). But make every effort to have these sex talks when they come up, and admit to discomfort and difficulties when you face them. Working through the trouble spots together will result in you and your lover feeling closer and more powerfully connected.

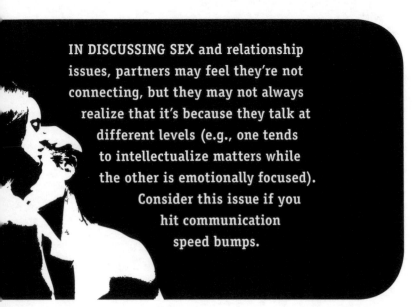

IN DISCUSSING SEX and relationship issues, partners may feel they're not connecting, but they may not always realize that it's because they talk at different levels (e.g., one tends to intellectualize matters while the other is emotionally focused). Consider this issue if you hit communication speed bumps.

Sexual Compatibility

After one or several date night discussions, you and your partner may have learned that you're two peas in a pod. Fantastic! Research confirms that the more alike lovers are, the greater their satisfaction with the relationship. This is in large part because similarity makes for far fewer conflicts. Many couples will find, however, that they don't see eye-to-eye on everything, including erotic talk and making sexy sounds, as Ruthie shares: "Well, the noise is pretty fun, but I think if you are mismatched with your partner, it can be a problem. My significant other and I are on opposite ends of the noisy spectrum, and I think sometimes it can keep us from being in the same place during sex."

If you find that you're not on the same page with your lover, rest assured there are ways to move forward together. Here's what you need to do:

Discuss the importance of sex objectively. Talk about your hopes for your sexual relationship, without judgment and see where you may have common ground, even on an issue that seems divisive. For example, if one lover is a morning person while the other is a night owl, this incompatibility can impact the amount of sex they have. This couple should come up with a compromise or creative arrangement that allows for sexual intimacy and conserves their energy for it.

Highlight the strong points in your relationship. It's important to remember how you and your lover are similar and what is working really well in the relationship. This will put you in a positive frame of mind and give you confidence to resolve sticking points or areas of friction.

Recognize that everyone is unique. Individuals have their own sexual abilities, preferences, and ways to express them. As with any other life issue, this individuality should be respected. Don't make your partner feel guilty or like he or she needs to apologize when it comes to his or her libido, sexual desires, or sexual preferences.

Don't label each other. Society promotes sameness—and that applies to how we have sex. So when lovers don't fit a particular idea or aren't having sex in a conventional or mainstream way, they can be made to feel inadequate, dysfunctional, abnormal, deviant, or inhibited. Take care not to name-call with these.

Educate yourselves. There's a lot of misinformation out there when it comes to sexuality. Many people are in the dark about what certain types of sexual behaviors, interactions, and responses are all about. Become more informed so that you can make more educated decisions about pushing your level of comfort and exploring your full erotic potential.

Consider therapy if you're having trouble working out compatibility issues. Negative reactions like sulking, criticizing, or feeling agitated can lead to hostility, strain, anger, and even cruelty. These reactions are unproductive and often need to be sorted through with the help of a professional.

"I'll show you mine if you show me yours" has never sounded so good. Showcasing your sexuality—putting your wares and pleasure on display before an adoring audience—will deliver the rock-star sex you crave. You take center stage as you teach your lover about your body, your sexual responses, and what you like. Your goal is to provide your lover with knowledge that can be used to enhance sex, with "show me" turning to "do it to me" as your lover learns to take you on the ride of your life.

If you're the guide:

Give encouragement. Saying things like, "You're so money when you rub me here, and it's out of this world with this kind of rhythm. . . . Mmmm. . . ." Affirming what your lover does well or getting him or her revved for what's to come will help your partner to feel confident, valued, and inspired.

Accept compliments. Better yet, enjoy them!

If you're the audience:

Pay attention. It can be easy to get lost in the moment and forget that you're supposed to be actively learning and not merely watching. Yes, this is a fantasy come true, but your task will be to send your lover beyond his or her wildest dreams.

Express appreciation. Everyone responds well to positive feedback about themselves, "I've never seen you look so sexy. I can't wait to do that to you."

TIME: take your time

LUST-INDUCING LOCATION: your bed

MATERIALS: any enhancements you feel are necessary for an A+ performance

PEAKING POTENTIAL: 4.5—some lovers may feel a little stilted in the guided performance, but the peak pay-off will be 5 rating in the long-term

Showing admiration for your guide and a desire to please can encourage more intimate and honest sharing.

IF YOUR PARTNER doesn't take instruction particularly well, listen to Bella's advice: "Expressing what you want is a great way to get what you want, and if it's done in a sexy way it's much less like a lesson and they seem to enjoy it more. I think guys really respect it when a woman knows her body and feels comfortable enough to say what she wants. The key is to make them feel like they are pleasing you and not that you are correcting them. This is best done with getting more reactive when things are done right, plus making more noise!"

Ask for more. Be eager to learn. If you need clarification or would like something to be repeated, try a simple "Encore!"

You can conduct your scintillating show-and-tell in a couple of different ways. One is to masturbate in front of your partner to show the kinds of touch you like and need during intercourse. Another way is to give your lover gentle, encouraging suggestions during a sex act, such as oral sex, to help him or her deliver maximum pleasure.

If you invite your lover to be a voyeur as you masturbate, approach the first peep show from top and bottom, working your way to your core. Explain which erogenous zones get you going when they're played with, emphasizing those that get more of a reaction with a partner's participation: "My ears are very sensitive, which is why it's such a shame that I can't kiss them. Instead, I fantasize about you taking me from behind but starting with gentle kisses on each ear. . . ."

Take your time and pleasure your body by caressing, rubbing, and massaging key zones, teasing your way to your groin. As you visit your various hot spots, explain that you may not get to all of them in one session, but that you're up for an entire semester of private tutoring to make sure that all of your orgasmic triggers are attended to. As you play with each part, explain what makes it feel so good—the pressure, the motion, the rhythm, the temperature, the texture—before slipping into a sexual frenzy and losing yourself in the sensations.

If you choose to give your lover guidance as you join together in a sex act, your objective is to describe what's working (or not), and to offer suggestions for making things even better and more electrifying. Here's the type of constructive feedback that will help your lover satisfy you:

→ I like it when you . . .
→ Please slow down. I want to make this last.

→ I'd like to try . . .
→ That's a little too . . . I need it more like . . . Yes!
→ I need a rest.
→ It would be wonderful if you could touch me [there] using [this move or technique] and [this type] of pressure.
→ I'm not so keen on . . . but it feels amazing when you . . .
→ Ooo . . . Aaaah . . . Yes! That's good. . . .

Be sure to check your tone: It should be caring, supportive, in charge, and sexy. Anything sounding harsh or critical risks shutting down your communication—and with it, your opportunity for better sex. Also, don't forget the sound effects, especially as you and your partner get things right. Let out a deep-throated moan, or an "Ooh!" when the technique, rhythm, or pressure is making your temperature rise.

Whether you're guiding or being guided, be generous with compliments for your partner. These can include:

→ It makes me smile when you . . .
→ My favorite thing about watching you is . . .
→ It feels so good when you . . .
→ I love it when you . . .
→ You look so sexy when you . . .

No matter which type of sharing you chose, process the experience together. Each of you needs feedback to the following questions:

→ What was the experience like?
→ What would you have liked me to do differently?
→ What needed more attention?
→ What should we do differently next time?
→ What else would you like to know?

Sharing What Sexy Talk Means to You

You and your partner have shared your erotic talk preferences with each other, and now it's time to put your money where your mouth is.

As you dive in, stay open to the possibilities. Your partner may surprise you. You may surprise yourself. You may find, for example, that talking dirty is actually easier than sharing more intimate, personal feelings. On the flip side, sharing personal feelings during sex can help you release deeply felt emotions. The idea is to experiment and explore until you discover what types of and how much erotic talk serves to sexually enhance your relationship with your lover. Here's what Reilly learned: "Silence would drive me nuts, so at least we're not about that. My lover is a lot quieter than I am, though. If I encourage him, he'll moan or say how good it feels, but often he's quiet until he climaxes. I get excited when I hear my partner, so I wish he'd give me even just a little bit more."

Be mindful as you enter into the exciting world of sexy talk that just because something gets said doesn't mean it's a request. Daniel knows that the erotic banter between him and his lover is a form of sex play and nothing more: "It's all unwritten, but it's all understood that just because we say it doesn't mean we want to do it. Like my lover gets turned on by a little dirty talk about a threesome, but that doesn't mean we are going to actually do it."

The key balance is to keep an open mind while acknowledging and respecting boundaries, as Wynn knows: "I don't have any limits, but part of that is because I know I am much more liberated than my partner. I know she will not tolerate talk in a degrading tone. Slut and whore are not good words to use. Neither is any kind of degrading act of intimacy. Light bondage is okay. But degradation or forcing of any kind is off-limits always."

Every couple has their own style and preferences, so just be honest and clear with your partner about what you like and what's off-limits. Tristan and his lover have it worked out: "No pornographic words are allowed. We are also not to discuss being aroused by other people when we have sex. We've further negotiated that I like it if I get a little humiliation from her, especially while I masturbate. She, on the other hand, does not like to receive humiliation talk from me."

Finally, don't wear out your lover with pressure to be creative and attentive in talking sexy. Pace yourselves or, like Ross, you'll find yourselves exhausted: "My partner loves it when I talk sexy. But it can be draining because it often seems to involve me inventing lengthy descriptions of erotic scenarios that I have to come up with off the top of my head. I like talking sexy, but only when it is natural and not a forced type of conversation, which is what it feels like when she keeps wanting more and more."

For this exercise, you're going to talk sexy during sex—whether that means foreplay, mutual masturbation, oral sex, or intercourse. This can involve any kind of erotic talk so go with what feels best for you. What this exercise provides is a chance to brainstorm ideas and develop a plot or storyline as you ease into your first erotic exchange or advance your efforts to the next level.

And even if you've put a lot of thought into screenwriting, directing, and producing your plotline, some-times the best strategy is to abandon it. Listen to Andy: "If it seems scripted, forced or 'over-thunk,' don't do it. You seem contrived and disconnected." You want to go with the flow, like Loren: "We like talking with dirty words like 'cock,' 'cunt,' 'fuck,' etc., while we're in foreplay and having sex. Usually, though, we end up abandoning it because we're having so much fun in the act!"

In formulating your loose plan of action as a storyteller, consider these following tips:

Developing the Plot

→ If you need an icebreaker that invites humor, use a cliché like "Would you like some cream with that?"

→ Describe the current action: Notice his erection, her sex flush, hard nipples . . .

→ Bring attention to your state of arousal: "I'm so wet right now" or "I'm dying to have you push my thong aside and circle my clit 'til I gush."

→ Offer a compliment: "It's so sexy to see you disappear into me like that."

→ Describe what you're about to do: "I'm going to then slip my leg around your waist, and press into you hard as I clutch your cock. . . ."

TIME: 30+ minutes

LUST-INDUCING LOCATION: wherever you have sex

MATERIALS: none required

PEAKING POTENTIAL: 5

- → Be willing to beg: "Please. Oh, please baby. Bring it. Slide your throbbing hot _____ into that dripping wet _____ . Fill me up until I can't take it anymore."
- → Describe the fantasy you're imagining: "Then, as your dick slides into Keri, Tina is going to straddle me so that everyone's genitals are being devoured. . . ."
- → Tune into senses of taste, touch, sound, and smell: "Your scent is driving me insane—I have to have you now!"
- → Check in with your partner: "Feel that? Like that?"
- → Issue commands: "I want more. Harder, deeper."
- → Aim for a combination of playful, naughty, and sweet nothings: "You're so sexy." "You're gorgeous." "I love your body." "I love your tits." "Your pussy is so tight." "I could lick your breasts/finger you/eat you out for hours." "You're going to get spanked." "Have you been a bad girl?" "You're very naughty."

Delivering the Goods

- → Put energy behind your statement. Flat lines are for the dead.
- → Consider timing. Sexy talk tends to be sexier when it's slower. This builds anticipation and adds to the dramatic effect. In the heat of the moment, of course, your words can pick up speed if that's what feels natural.
- → Keep your voice volume low to create interest and intimacy.
- → Take advantage of circumstances that make your voice sound sexy, like morning voice. For example, I'm allergic to cigarettes, so if I've been in a smoky room, my voice gets lower and huskier, and, in turn, sexier. I try not to let that go to waste.
- → Perform the occasional sound check. What do you sound like? Should you make your voice softer, smoother, or more expressive, especially in your ooos, ahhs, and ohhs?

What follows is like a toolbox packed with hot and helpful quotes to say to your lover during sex. Pick out a few or try them all and see what works wonders!

Praise/Affirmations
→ That feels great!
→ Keep saying it that way.
→ I love it when you touch me there.
→ That feels amazing!
→ I love it when you hit that spot!
→ You know how to touch me just right.
→ You're so good at turning me on.
→ Oh, God!
→ That was the best yet!
→ That feels so delicious.
→ You feel so good.
→ Perfect!
→ That feels incredible—don't stop!
→ That was terrific!

Expressions of Attraction
→ I love your body.
→ You're so sexy.
→ You have the most gorgeous . . .
→ I can't believe how beautiful you are.

→ You look so hot right now.
→ I love the way you're looking at me right now.
→ I love the way you smell.
→ I love seeing you react that way.
→ I'm crazy about you.
→ I can't concentrate on anything else right now.

Heartfelt Sentiments
→ You're so precious to me.
→ I cherish you so much.
→ I love you with all my heart.
→ I love you so much it hurts.
→ You are the love of my life.
→ I need you like the air I breathe.
→ I've never held anyone as beautiful as you.
→ I'm head over heels for you.
→ I feel so . . . /You feel so . . .
→ I love your . . . /being . . .

→ It feels so good to have your arms around me.
→ You feel so good in my arms.
→ I feel at peace when I'm sleeping next to you.
→ Thank you for . . .

→ I can't wait to hold you in my arms.

→ I want to make love to you.

Desire

→ I'd love it if you'd . . .

→ I can't get enough of you.

→ I've been thinking about you all day

→ I want to merge with you.

→ I'd love to lick your . . .

→ I'd love to cum all over your . . .

→ I can't wait to feel you inside me.

→ You look ravishing right now.

→ You know what I'd like from you now more than anything?

→ I want to savor you/your . . .

Appreciating Moments

→ It's so much fun to have sex with you.

→ Give me more.

→ You have such a sweet . . .

→ Your lips taste so good

→ I love your touch.

→ Your skin is so soft and smooth.

→ You feel so good against me.

→ Your hand feels so good in mine.

→ You belong inside me.

→ I love it when you play with my hair.

Observations

→ I can feel you getting . . .

→ You're getting me hard.

→ You're turning me on.

→ I love how hard you are.

→ You're so wet right now.

→ I can feel the sensation spreading through me.

→ I get aroused when you moan like that.

→ The way you're looking at me right now has me so . . .

Commands

→ Feel me.

→ Tease my . . .

→ Grab my . . .

→ Give it to me hard now.

→ Tell me about your . . .

→ Open your legs.

→ Now ask me for another.

Questions

→ What do you want me to do right now?

→ What do you need from me the most?

→ How can I excite you?

→ How do you like that?

→ Do you want some more?

→ You want some of this?

Dirty Talk

→ I'm going to put you over my knee and spank you hard.

→ Want me to wrap my wet lips around your rock-hard cock?

→ I'm going to stuff that big hard prick in to my slippery wet . . .

→ I'm gonna put my pulsating dick in your tight, hot pussy.

→ Spread your sweet ass for my cock.

→ Bend me over and yank my panties down around my ankles.

→ I'm going to spread your legs and . . .

→ I want to fuck you right now.

→ I want you to fuck me.

→ I want your hand on my . . .

→ Grab my ass!

→ Make my . . .

→ I want you to_____ my . . .

→ I want to_____ your . . .

→ Thinking about you makes my . . .

→ I want to play with your . . .

→ I want to make your . . .

→ I love the way your _____ feels against my . . .

RESEARCH HAS FOUND that men find women who speak in a higher-pitched voice attractive.

Chapter 3 Check-In

You've just invested quality time learning how to react to each other and encouraging more sexual sharing. You're opening up when it comes to achieving mutual pleasuring. And you just gave one hell of a sex show. In measuring if you've reached the place you want to be, consider these questions:

→ What worked during your discussions, sharing, and providing feedback? What didn't?

→ Are there additional or different rules of engagement that would've made your talks easier and more successful?

→ Are there topics you want to revisit, including any compatibility issues? Are there topics that were missing from the list?

→ What could you do differently to improve discussions? What do you hope your partner will or won't do the next time you have a talk?

→ What was it like to share your body with your lover in a whole different way?

→ How was the erotic talk? What would you try again, perhaps with a twist? What didn't work at all? Which type of erotic talk would you be up for next time? How did attempts at dirty talk go?

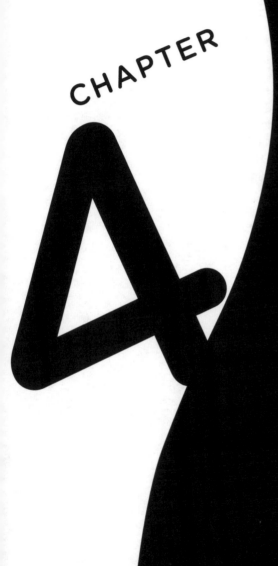

Firing Up Foreplay:
Scenarios to Heat Up the Bedroom

IN CHAPTER 4, YOU'LL LEARN HOW TO:

- ✔ Sex up seduction scenarios using erotic talk.

- ✔ Add some serious body talk to your flirting and seduction efforts!

- ✔ Get tips for erotic talk during afterplay.

"I'm going to devour you when I get home." "Your scent is driving me mad." "You're going to lose it when you see the lacy get-up I slipped into for our date. Wanna peek?" "Mmmm . . . I've been missing these lips all day!" "I can't wait to get you home and fuck you." "Have I mentioned I'm quite flexible?"

PEOPLE DELIVER EROTIC TALK in all sorts of ways all day. Now that you have a better sense of the different ways people can dish out fantasy-fueling fodder, you can, in essence, have sex 24/7 should you desire.

Starting with an early morning romp, breaking for a midday quickie, and culminating in a late night roll in the hay, you can stretch the limits of your sex life. Seems inconceivable? Not when you think about sex entailing far more than intercourse. Foreplay, for one, is a critical part of sexual trysts and affairs. Many women—and men—need to be erotically stimulated before they respond to a lover's "Let's make love" or beg someone to "Fuck my brains out!" So open your mind—and loins—to what it would be like to engage in 'round-the-clock love sessions.

The best kind of foreplay, the kind that yields the best results, is an all-day, everyday affair that inspires lovers to seek out more sensational sex. With this kind of "work" play, it's easy to take things from sleepy to scintillating in the blink of an eye by using the aural to your advantage. Sexy talk is mental foreplay, and lovers know that what-you-say seduction is what sets animalistic appetites ablaze. Partners become salivating sensualists as they lose themselves in the energy, lust, and anticipation of pursuing or being fervently pursued.

So in this chapter, we'll focus on using your mouth to drive foreplay. (Note: While we touch on phone sex here, chapter 5 goes into depth about all the remote ways both of you can get trussed up with technology.) We're also going to incorporate some naughty nonverbal communication in bringing lovers to their knees: body talk. We express a great deal of our desires and desirability through body language and facial expressions. Just like a well-coordinated dance, we want you to wow your audience by fluidly showcasing your sexual gestures, body stance, and movements. Doing so amplifies what you're saying to your lover for a finishing touch that gets you more touch.

Becoming Flirtalicious

Whether you and your partner have been together forever or just met, flirting should be a consistent part of your sexual repertoire. Teasing, enamoring "play with me" innuendos can ignite a thirst that's never quenched if you're clever about this passion prelude. So we're going to explore how you can stealthily sprinkle some spice into your daily—and nightly—routine. In no time, you will have your lover nibbling at your forbidden fruits.

Everyone loves a good flirt, and good flirts reap the benefits from their abilities. Listen to Adam: "Throwing out random sex talk outside of sexual situations, but seriously, and not in a facetious way, always gives a little jolt of sexual energy to a day that can lead to thinking about sex, and then being horny later on." It's the ultimate ego boost as lovers rev their sexual engines, charming and charging each other up in a foreplay that engages mind, body, and heart. They become friskier, sexier, warmer, and more lovable, open, and adventurous. So here we're all about making you absolutely irresistible at every hour and stage of the game.

SITUATION: FORGET-ME-NOT SEND-OFF

What It Calls For: Go beyond the old-fashioned morning pucker up.
Body Talk: The original meaning of flirt was "a brief glance," so give your lover

a sexy, mischievous look as you slip a note into his or her pocket. Then give him or her a lingering, you'll-want-to-come-back-for-more kiss before planting a firm pat on the rear as your partner heads for the door.

Erotic Talk Recommendations: Your forget-me-not note should be simple, along the lines of:

YOU'RE IN LUCK if your lover is an auditory type—a person who is mostly connected to the world through sound/silence and hearing/listening. About 20 percent of individuals fall into this category: They are sensitive to music, affectionate statements, and whether a sound is good or not. The very tone of your voice can draw them in and open them up, so use this to your advantage.

→ "You make me so happy. And I plan to make you *very* happy later."

→ "You make my heart skip a beat."

→ "I want to _____ your _____ as soon as you come home, you/my_____." (You fill in the blanks, making it as romantic or wash-your-mouth-out-with-soap dirty as you like.)

From the moment you wake up, you want to groom yourselves for getting it on later. You can start with things like "I love waking up with you" or "You look so handsome in that." Then keep the compliments coming throughout the day: "Hey sexy thing! Just wanted to let you know that I'm thinking about you" or "I can almost feel myself wrapped around you."

SITUATION: LUSTING-FOR-YOU LUNCH BREAK

What It Calls For: Fill your lover in on the uncensored version of "thinking of you."

Body Talk: You need to describe your devilish daydreams since your lover is probably not with you.

Erotic Talk Recommendations: Your goal is to make your lover feel that you'd rather be home playing hookie, tending to life's most important thing—your significant other. This can be as straightforward as "I so wish I was with you now" or "I can't wait to make love to you later," or it can veer toward the obscene, "I'm unzipping my pants, thinking about your rampant cock . . . ," "I'm imagining myself plunging into you and it's really turning me on . . . ," "I'm being such a naughty girl with my lipstick vibe. Hope my boss doesn't catch me!"

SITUATION: HORNY AS HELL

What It Calls For: Have witty, playful conversation that teases the mind to the point that your partner can hardly be contained and must have a quickie. Tor can tell you: "Once when she told me about wanting or needing me to take her, I rushed home from work and took her aggressively. All the while talking to her, telling her how I was going to take her, how I was going to please myself with her. She really liked that."

Body Talk: You're hot, sweaty, and out of breath. What more needs to be said?

Erotic Talk Recommendations: Start with things like, "I've been thinking about you all day," "I'd love to lick your _____ right now," "I'd love to cum all over your . . . ," or "I want to make you . . . " In kicking off your quickie quest, show up with something like, "So you wanna play?" or "It sounded like you need a good fuck."

SITUATION: FLUSHED IN THE MIDDLE OF RUSH HOUR

What It Calls For: Have "talk to me" rush-hour action that puts the likes of Aphrodite to shame.

Body Talk: Full disclosure is needed because your lover can't see you.

Erotic Talk Recommendations: "I've got such a raging hard-on right now." "I'm flexing my vajayjay, thinking of what it's going to be like to have you glide between my lips."

Some people go one step further, adding a layer of foreplay *before* the foreplay, like Samuli: "I work best by setting up a situation where we are already dialed in to each other, then playing into that dynamic. My partner loves it when I have a gig—when I'm playing in a bar—and I talk dirty to her on a set break, and then look at her when I go back on stage. I don't think the dirty talk can really stand completely alone." Erotic talk on the way home from work can redirect the day's carnal communication efforts to the express lane to XXX action once you're home. Here's what Kai had to say: "My partner sometimes calls as she's driving home from work, and things often quickly turn to phone sex. She is then so ready to go when she gets home and loves that I'm there, already naked and on the bed, waiting for her to make it all come true."

SITUATION: VERY HAPPY HOUR

What It Calls For: Become a superflirt by combining body talk with lascivious lip action. It has huge pay offs, as Nic can attest: "Sitting in a bar, I explained to her what I was going to do to her, combining both explicit and general phrases. . . . Her pupils dilated, her lips parted, and her breathing got ragged. I left money on the table, stood, put out my hand, and said, 'Let's go.' She did."

Body Talk: This is your chance to flirt like a champ. Cozy up to the bar, order drinks, and plan your personal sexy soiree, adding to the sizzle by:

→ Maintaining eye contact to engage your lover, but not before allowing your lips to part for a moment as you begin to gaze into each other's eyes. Locking eyes is a way of showing interest and entering each other's personal zones.

RESEARCH HAS FOUND that heterosexual women at a singles' bar exhibit far more nonverbal displays directed at men than the other way around. Ironically, while men tend to think that they're taking the initiative, they are actually responding to women's nonverbal overtures, like glancing behaviors, nodding, smiling, and laughing.

- Showing that you're into this time together with your facial expressions—for example, by raising your eyebrows in reaction to a sexy sentiment and giving the occasional head nod to acknowledge what is building between you.
- Closing the gap between you and your date by perching on the edge of your seat and giving little, light touches on your date's arm or knee.
- Tilting your head to the side to show that you like your date.
- Head-tossing, hair flipping, or hair fiddling to further indicate sexual interest.

Erotic Talk Recommendations: Greet each other with a warm hug and a kiss and something like, "You look so adorable, I could eat you up—and might just have to later," or "Just thinking about seeing you was turning me on."

Note: Your honey might not be into public displays of affection, or PDAs. Do what feels right for both of you. For example, Hoda has her boundaries: "Unspoken rules are not to become sexual in front of others, unless it's a secret signal or word." Situations like these make urgent whispers of wanting all the more necessary! So speak softly and sexy, banking on some sonorous surround sound later.

SITUATION: A PRE-NOOKIE NIGHT ON THE TOWN

What It Calls For: Have bold wordplay along the lines of "You're such a cock/cunt tease." There's nothing like it, as Jesse knows: "She was dressed very sexy and we were out for the evening, and I knew that she had nothing on underneath her dress. We did the dinner and movie, then went out for drinks, and I was touching her and feeling her all night, practically everywhere we went. Part of the fun was knowing that others were sneaking peeks and enjoying watching us.

Body Talk: Building upon your hot 'n heavy happy hour, practice postural echoing, in which you mirror each other's breathing, talking, body postures, facial expressions, and head movements for better synergy. Mimicry is a form of flattery and helps people feel more connected. You can further boost your sexual electricity with these tactics:

→ Stroke the length of your neck or caress the back of your calf while smiling demurely and making eye contact.

→ Run your fingers through your hair.

→ Fiddle with the buttons on your shirt.

These touches indicate where you might want to be stroked later. Just make sure to pace yourselves so you

RESEARCH HAS FOUND that women are typically more aware than men of what's going on during a flirtation, making note of a man's interest in the way he moves, dances, and looks at her. Men aren't as focused on the subtleties of how a woman handles herself to gauge her interest. Instead, they look for clues in what she does to demonstrate her interest—for instance, allowing him to buy her a drink.

don't skip the restaurant, movie theater, or night club. Transmitting sexual sparks at a public space ups the ante, as Audrey well knows: "When out, and if I'm wearing a certain type of get-up, then we have this thing that we do every now and then. He whispers in my ear that he knows I am not wearing panties—that he wants to slide his fingers in and out of my wet pussy while at dinner or wherever we're at. I can't help but smile at memories of him inserting his fingers slowly and everyone wondering why the big smiles. It is erotic because he and I are the only ones in the room who know what is going on." I wouldn't bet on that, Audrey, but obviously no one is complaining.

Erotic Talk Recommendations: As you make your moves, allow yourself to get more romantic, seductive, or down-right dirty with lines like: "You have an unbelievable body," "I thought we'd start with you screwing my tits, then my mouth, then my pussy," "I can't wait to be inside you," or "I need to have you naked."

SITUATION: DIRTY DANCING

What It Calls For: All of your best moves. Dance is a fantastic way to release your energy, including sexual energy, and is pretty much guaranteed to put you and your lover in a happier, more playful mood for loving. Katja is a big fan: "Dancing makes everything all the more heated, and the sex—it becomes more savage and passionate at the same time."

Body Talk: Brush against each other's skin as you twirl, bend, or lead the other. Slowly lick your lips with a half-curled smile and wink when your eyes meet. Moist lips and a flushed face will boost your lover's adrenaline and heart rate, increasing his or her desire to have you even more!

Erotic Talk Recommendations: There's not much that needs to be said if you're lost in a dance together, but if you want to whisper something, consider the type of dance you're doing. Dirty dancing—"I was thinking how you'll get me all hot 'n sweaty later, too"—may summon something completely differ-ent from, say, a romantic slow dance—"You own this room, my love. All eyes are on you."

SITUATION: GETTING FRESH AT A LATE NIGHT FÊTE

What It Calls For: Become bold with your lover—above and beyond a little PDA—especially if you get busted.

Body Talk: Kissing, caressing, and possibly escaping to a bathroom or abandoned room for some hot play—the trick to luring your partner in is lowering your voice so that he or she has to lean close to hear you. Then the full-on seduction begins with the kind of erotic talk that lets your lover know what's on your mind.

Erotic Talk Recommendations: I'm going to let Sam take this one: "I tend to love to be verbally dominated, but in a sweet way. I had a younger lover (he was thirty; I was forty eight) who was good at the 'mind fuck.' . . . We'd be at a party and he'd whisper, 'I know you're thinking about my cock in your pussy, aren't you? You can't wait to let me in there. . . .' I melt over that kind of talk. When we would be alone, he whispered more of the same, 'Oh you're such a good girl. You love to give it all up for me,' or 'You'd fuck every guy in the room for me if I told you to, wouldn't you?'—things that played on my submissive nature and his dominant side."

SITUATION: PROTECTING WHILE PUMPING UP PASSION

What It Calls For: Have honest communication, believing that safer sex can make for some of the hottest sex.

Body Talk: Reach for the condom, dental dam (latex or plastic wrap barrier placed over vulva or anus during sexual activity), or latex glove.

Erotic Talk Recommendations: Protect yourself against unwanted pregnancy and sexually transmitted infections by saying things like "Let's put a rubber on that perfect prick of yours so that you can slide into my . . . ," "I'm going to squeeze some of this silky smooth lube into the tip of this condom so that you feel my every move" (for condoms); "I can't wait to spread my legs and have you lube me up for some fine-dining, bon-appetit action" (for dental dams); or "I love playing doctor. Nurse, could you please put on my gloves?" (for latex gloves).

SITUATION: CIRCLING THE CHERRY

What It Calls For: Perform some serious tongue action.

Body Talk: If you are the giver, after you've warmed her up, take your time brushing the inner lips of her vulva with your lips, then lick upward along each side as you tenderly spread her labia to expose her clitoris. Warm up her "cherry" with kisses before fluttering the tip of your tongue across it. You can also take it into your mouth to gently caress it with your tongue, slowly circling it and working up your pace and the intensity of your pressure. Stroke her thighs or caress her breasts as your mouth and tongue work their magic.

If you're the receiver, guide your partner by giving feedback about the pressure, pace, and kinds of stimulation you want. As your partner performs cunnilingus on you, you can add more enthusiasm to the action or heighten the sensation by pressing your pelvis into your partner's mouth and riding the tongue or squeezing your thighs around your partner's head (taking care not to overdo it).

Erotic Talk Recommendations: If you're the giver, let her know how eager you are to go down on her: "I want to lick you until you come!" "I want to bury myself between your legs." Once you're having at her, keep up the verbal vigor: "I love the way you taste!" "Oh God, your scent is intoxicating." If you and your lover are still getting to know each other, it's always a good idea to check in: "Am I too rough?" "Do you like it faster?" "Would you prefer less pressure?"

If you're the receiver, your body talk—squirming, writhing, arching—says a lot. But don't stop there; let yourself moan, gasp, scream, cry out—whatever comes from your core as your lover works up a luscious lather. Give positive feedback: "Oh yeah, I'm loving how you're licking it. Make me cum!" "I love it when you eat me out." "God, you're insatiable!" When necessary, provide some direction: "I want more of that!" "Oh baby, I can't take any more there but would love it if you'd. . . ."

SITUATION: GIVING HEAD

What It Calls For: Open wide.

Body Talk: Not everyone is a "deep throat" fan, so be careful not to get carried away while your lover goes down on you. An easy, shallow thrusting or circling of the hips is usually okay—any more than that calls for checking in with your lover to make sure he or she is okay.

Erotic Talk Recommendations: If you are the giver, take the time to admire his genitalia. For example, fondle his balls while murmuring "Niiiiiice," or stroke his shaft while saying, "You are so fine." Naturally, your erotic talk efforts will take place before going south since your mouth will then be full, so have fun teasing and flattering before taking his penis into your mouth: "It's time for you to get your reward." "Mmm, I'm so in the mood to suck cock."

As you take him into your mouth as deeply and fully as you like, moan like you're dying of hunger and begin to mimic a thrusting action. Caress the shaft with your tongue and lips, sucking on it as if you might swallow it. Use your hands to massage, stroke, or gently squeeze his scrotum and inner thighs. If you want feedback at any point, withdraw for a moment while stroking the shaft and ask, "Do you like the rhythm?" "Want my lips tighter?" "Does it hurt you if I teabag you? I want to get all over your sac with some sucking action."

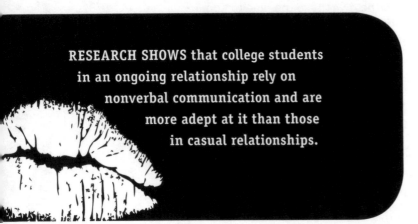

RESEARCH SHOWS that college students in an ongoing relationship rely on nonverbal communication and are more adept at it than those in casual relationships.

If you're the receiver, give your partner guidance on the pressure, pace, and kinds of touches that get your juices flowing. Tell your partner if you're nearing orgasm and would like to transition to another position or activity. If your partner doesn't want you to ejaculate in his or her mouth, give an advance warning. More than anything, get vocal. Lovers crave this kind of affirmation. They want to know when something feels amazing. It can be as simple as, "That feels incredible!" or "Ohh, this is perfect."

SITUATION: INVITE-ONLY TOY PARTY

What It Calls For: Host a private sex party complete with the vibrating sex toys of your choice.

Body Talk: Any indicator that your body is aroused and sexually responding works here: an erection, the appearance of pre-cum, vaginal lubrication, a sex flush, hard nipples. . . .

Erotic Talk Recommendations: When sampling a product, provide feedback on how it feels: "It feels really good there like that." "It's a bit uncomfortable." "Let's crank it up more." "I can't handle that kind of vibration." "I'm so glad that I'm sharing this with you." "I'm having so much fun." "There's nothing like it." "What can I do to make it feel even better?"

Have fun playing and pleasuring with your toys, but it's important to reassure your lover that he or she couldn't possibly be replaced by a piece of plastic or a battery-powered gadget: "Nothing pleasures me like you do." "I like this, but I hunger for you."

SITUATION: MÉNAGE À TROIS

What It Calls For: Discuss everything ahead of time.

Body Talk: Everything we've discussed, only times two.

Erotic Talk Recommendations: Having a threesome involves a great deal of sex communication, relying on skills you learned in chapter 3. Sure, threesome opportunities can pop up unexpectedly, and you may feel like you can deal with things later. But as anybody who has had a threesome will tell you, lovers need to talk about issues, especially if you're part of a couple roping in a third party. It's wise to discuss the following topics ahead of time:

1. What are your fantasies around threesomes? What turns you on and off about them?
2. Do you want a situation where one person watches the other two, like a voyeur? Or were you thinking that everybody would pleasure each other at the same time? Or a bit of both? Or would everybody only masturbate?
3. Do you expect any pairing off? Is that okay?
4. What's your safer sex plan?
5. How will you manage unexpected jealous feelings? Can your relationship handle them?
6. You need to be prepared for feelings such as doubt or inadequacy that can arise. The best way to do this is by having open, honest communication.

Amorous Afterplay

Regardless of your pregame erotic exertions, there's no better nightcap following the main event than time well spent luxuriating in sounds and affirmations, like Lindsey does: "We tell each other often, postgame, what we liked, how something was, how great it was, etc., like, 'You really sucked my cock well' or 'I loved it when you used two fingers.' It sort of extends the electricity we just generated."

In addition to sighs of contentment and other vocal affirmations, you could say any of the following:

→ "I take it you enjoyed yourself?"
→ "Hold me."
→ "You're such an amazing fuck."
→ "Let's do it again!"
→ "That really meant a lot."
→ "I'm so glad I got to share that with you."
→ "Sweet dreams, astounding one."

Sharing this downtime together will make you feel closer, strengthening your connection and the emotions you have for one another. Such afterplay also offers up heartfelt appreciation, which may get your lover primed for another round. . . .

Chapter 4 Check-In

For this chapter, we relied on hot lips and suggestive body language when becoming mad flirts to lure and land your partner. Process what you learned by considering these questions:

1. What did you like about your efforts? What were some of the highlights?
2. What didn't fly? Is it something that can be fixed or is it out of the question for now?
3. How did it feel to be flirt shamelessly and play up your body talk?
4. What kind of flirting opportunities would you like to set up in the future?
5. What types of sounds and utterances do you want to hear the next time you play with each other?
6. What sexy scenarios or foreplay inspirations do you hope to execute in the future that you've dreamt up all on your own?

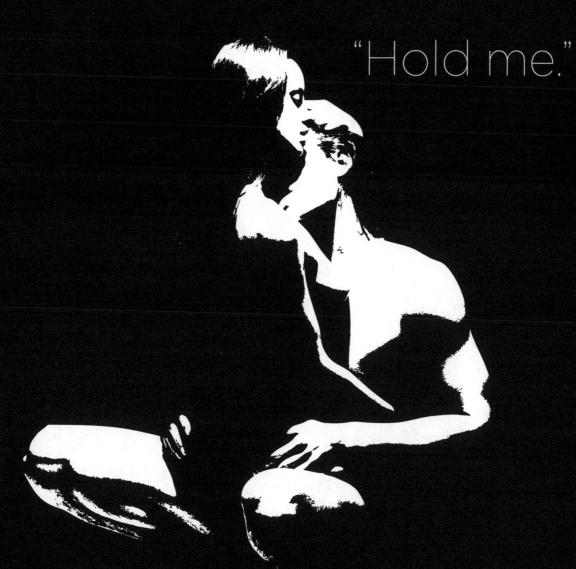

"Hold me."

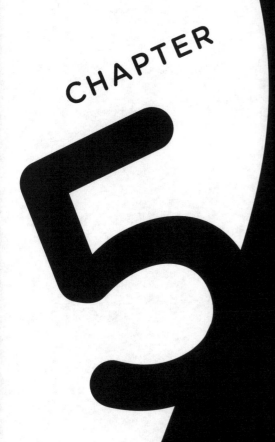

CHAPTER

5

Erotic Talk Tech-Style:
Seduce Your Partner Via Email, Texts, and More

IN CHAPTER 5, YOU'LL LEARN HOW TO:

☞ Draft delectable emails.

☞ Master the rules of tech-style erotic engagement.

☞ Win over your beau with text messages.

☞ Discover the erotic freedom of instant messaging.

☞ Skillfully intrigue by using the many forms of cybersex.

☞ Become accomplished in the art of aural phone sex.

Can't wait 4 2nite. Outfit = easy access. ;o)

M drooling. GTH4U. *(Got the hots for you.)*

M about 2 step in2 the shower. Wish u
were here.
Me 2. Luv 2 get u all dirty then sudsy.
M already dripping wet.

IN OR OUT OF THE BEDROOM, nothing heats up your sex life like making seduction an all-day affair. You're both bound to get off in arousing each other with naughty notes or scintillating sounds that plant the seeds for good times to come. Familiar and anonymous e-lovers delight in sending mind-blowing missives, opening a passion-filled Pandora's box of vivid visuals and libidinal stirs that keep both hungering for more. Teasing your flirt to no end via sexy emails, text messages, instant messages, cybersex, and phone sex can trigger some of your hottest sexual escapades, upping the arousal ante before you've even touched.

In fueling each other's sexual energy and building anticipation, you fill sex-starved moments with thoughts of impure pleasure and adventure, as Debra describes: "My partner and I are workaholics and don't see each other nearly enough. So we need to tap every means of communication around, and the hotter the better. While we may be out of sight, we're on the other's mind. Constantly flirtexting or sexting is part of our staying power. We're still head over heels for each other and ready to get all over each other when the opportunity presents itself."

Whether near or far, tech sex takes foreplay to a whole new level. Lovers can become so aroused from their bold banter that sparks are already flying by the time they finally meet. Tech sex also helps lovers explore new frontiers, as Sidney explains: "Using different forms of technology, like text messages and emails, has been a great way to ease into [erotic talk,] an area my partner has been slow to embrace. We're being almost naughty, but somehow it's allowed. The exchanges are distant enough to be exciting without interrupting the flow [she's comfortable with] in the bedroom ."

With every new communication gadget, lovers are quickly figuring out how to reach out and "touch" each other for sexual thrills. Those looking for action have embraced tech sex as a way to meet and get acquainted with others interested in sex or love online. Tara explains: "It's huge. I've met most of my sex partners online, so that's how it begins. The barriers are broken down much more quickly with technology. I don't know if that's always such a good thing overall, but I enjoy breaking those barriers and using my cell phone for texting sexy messages and sometimes pictures, and emails have become erotic novellas."

Tech sex is evolving daily. So far, your menu of erotic options includes what is outlined in the following sections.

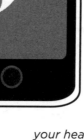

Eye-Popping, Eros-Inducing Emails

Hey sexy—Have been trying to get some work done, but am having trouble concentrating. Is it any wonder that I'm a bit distracted given the visions I'm having about us? Mmm . . . like . . . my red-hot mouth making its way down your treasure trail . . . your fingers racing over my scantily covered curves, hungry for my slippery, inviting hole . . . sending tremors through your body as my lips grip your hard cock, my tongue doing its magic . . . working your swollen, aching member between my thighs, my crotch dripping, drooling for a taste of you . . . hearing you moan as you remove my damp g-string with your teeth, your head bobbing madly between my legs . . . whimpering as I please your every whim . . .

Whether you aim to tease, torment, or seduce, sexy email is where it's at when it comes to XXX-treme e-flirting.

This erotic message elicited quite the reaction from my then-long-distance lover—so much so that I used it years later with another boyfriend, and not surprisingly, my cock-teasing made him equally randy. (There's nothing wrong with recycling your own "juice" on occasion, especially if it's too good not to replay.)

Sexy emails have become the erotic elixir of our times. Many people even post "wanted" adverts on websites like Craigslist, hoping to find someone who is game for an online tryst. Instigating online dirty dealings with a beau or partner can benefit your relationship because they:

Serve to sexually excite. Erotic emails set sexual arousal in motion, increasing your desire for one another and helping you get in the mood. Lusty lingo further helps in holding you over 'til the next time you can see each other.

Bolster your mood. Being regularly reminded that you're absolutely irresistible—that someone can't wait to get all over you—is a powerful ego boost that can energize your body, mind, and soul.

Empower. Writing suggestive sentiments is sometimes able to coax anyone reserved or reluctant into some carnal conversation. Safe from afar, you can take your time crafting your own ravenous response to a lover's expression of "can't resist you" cravings. Those who feel that the written word is their most effective means of communication will embrace these tit-for-tat titillations with the knowledge that they're in their erotic element during these exchanges.

Induce fantasies. Erotic emails set the stage for scenarios you can play out later. They're also an excellent way for shy or silent lovers to introduce ideas they may not otherwise suggest. Assuming a screenwriter's guise, they can test the waters, writing about imagined encounters that a lover may be excited about exploring.

Keep the romance and passion alive. Couples who are mindful about tantalizing each other throughout the week via email encourage a vibrant, dynamic sex life. Their inbox becomes a constant reminder of why they fell for each other and why they still hunger for more. By sending affectionate and erotic emails, lovers demonstrate to one another that their relationship and sexual needs are top priority.

Van couldn't agree more: "The occasional dirty text or email message throughout the day can turn the afternoon blahs into something to look forward to when I get home. It allows for more communication and passion-building suspense."

Drafting Something Delectable

Perhaps the most intimidating thing about sexy emails is what to say. Step one is realizing that very few people are born erotica writers, so cut yourself some slack. Step two is knowing that you don't have to compose a romance novel. Your lover will be thrilled if you:

➔ Send love quotes.
➔ Write a passion-filled poem.
➔ Email a song with meaningful lyrics.
➔ Copy a steamy passage from an erotic anthology (look for collections edited by Alison Tyler, for example).

➔ Recall and describe something you did with—or without—this partner. (After all, "write what you know" is the first bit of advice given to aspiring writers.)

Remember, it's more than okay to borrow inspiration from published sources. Just get in tune with your lover's tastes and give credit where credit's due if you're quoting someone famous. For example, Rumi, a thirteenth century Persian poet, is well-known for his inspirational works. Consider this excerpt:

In the orchard and rose garden,

I long to see your face. In the taste of sweetness, I long to kiss your lips. In the shadows of passion, I long for your love.

It would be a bit cheeky for your lover to come across Rumi's writings elsewhere, like on a subway advertisement (which I have seen), only to realize that you plagiarized. So always cite your sources.

If you're determined to be original, go for it, and any lover worthy of your efforts will be won over by your initiative and amorous attempts—and hopefully respond in kind.

Here are three basic steps to follow when drafting your eros-inducing email:

1. Decide if your emails are going to be written in the first or third person. Are they going to be about what you're doing (or at least wish you were doing) at this very moment or later that night? Or are you interesting in creating a scene involving a hypothetical couple that represents the two of you?

2. Focus on your partner's allure and desirability, at least in the first couple of messages. What makes your lover so attractive? What turns you on? What do you long to touch, kiss, fondle, lick? People can never hear enough flattering things about themselves, so play it up. The more a person is made to feel attractive, the greater his or her sexual responsiveness.

3. Cater to your partner's preferences, at least in the beginning. For example, if she's into spanking, describe how you plan to get her on all fours before licking your hand for a nice, wet sting.

From here on out, what you write depends on how your partner responds. In maintaining the momen-tum, try to abide by the following guidelines in setting your hearts (and loins) aflutter:

1. Respond sooner rather than later. Nothing can be more agonizing than waiting—and waiting—for someone to play with you in this way. Not only did your lover make him or herself vulnerable by writing a naughty note, but he or she wants confirmation that your interest has been piqued. So it's your job to acknowledge a lover's attempts at e-sex ASAP.

2. When you respond to your partner, highlight what you liked most about the e-mail. This encourages more of what worked and weeds out anything that was a turn-off.

3. Ask questions. They keep the dialogue going and build the "plot." Questions also show that you're most intrigued by what's going on.

Remember, in exchanging sexy emails, you're basically building a story together. Framing this sexual adventure as such makes it less intimidating, allowing for twists and turns, and positions that may not have been imagined otherwise. As you write your sex saga, strive to use as many descriptors as possible. Suggestions like the following will hold your lover's attention more than anything: "I want to be making slow, sin-tillating love to your deliciously sexy body, my tongue tickling your lips as we roll around in my soft, warm bed, working up a sweat as I go deeper and deeper into all of your holes. . . ."

Just be clear and direct about what you want. The challenge when it comes to any kind of e-correspondence is making sure the reader can interpret the intended tone. A study commissioned by Microsoft Canada found that one in three email users have had an email misinterpreted. Complicating matters further, research has found that a person has a fifty-fifty chance of ascertaining the tone of an email message. Since your lover cannot read your body language and can't see your facial expressions, make sure to reread what you've typed, asking, "How would I interpret this if it was sent to me?" For emphasis and flourish, try using the emoticons, such as :) or ;) or <3 , or capital letters to get your intent across.

RULES OF ENGAGEMENT

Before signing off from sexy emails, there are a few important don'ts to highlight. After all, you don't want to sabotage your amorous efforts:

1. Do *not* send erotic messages to or from a work email. Big Brother is watching and will frown on your real and imagined sexual exploits. In the same vein, consider where your sweetie will be when the sexy email is received. Even if your lover has a nonwork account, some work spaces do not provide sufficient privacy for this kind of "sexchange."

2. Unless you know your lover craves it, refrain from being too vulgar. Men, in particular, have been criticized for going overboard in this way. A

classic example: "I'm slapping my meat, thinking about you." Such slang may work with the guys, but it's probably not going to evoke "Yeah, baby!" from gals.

3. Think twice before engaging in erotic exchanges with a casual or new lover or an online acquaintance. E-thrills require a different degree of trust than personal communications. A person whose loyalty to you has yet to be proven may find it amusing to share your writings—and who knows what kind of damage that can do.

4. Piggybacking on the trust issue, unless you've already exchanged explicit emails, wait until you've gotten to know your partner well to do so. Some lovers are not receptive to pornographic play until they're quite comfortable with the relation-ship. It's safer to start with romantic expressions or sensual innuendos, working your way up to more graphic suggestions if that's what you are both hot for.

5. Avoid clichés; you'll sound cheesy: "If I were to lay eleven roses next to you, you'd make the perfect dozen."

It's easy to presume that technology is your fast pass to no-holds-barred sex from afar. It may seem like everyone is typing away with this wildly popular technology, writing lines that would make a trucker blush. But that's not so. "Anything goes" may work for some couples, but others must play it smart, like Joelle and her beau: "We don't exchange erotic emails. There are too many hackers out there, and his is the kind of career that would end over such exchanges being uncovered. My job is a bit more liberal, but if I'm exposed, he's exposed. He signs his emails either 'L' (which is short for 'love'), or the French 'Je t'aime,' but never 'love' or 'I love you', etc. He saves that for good old-fashioned missives."

Joelle brings up a great point—taking the old-fashioned route. There's a long tradition of lovers exchanging lurid letters. The fact that they've become the exception to the rule—that they require extra effort to write—is sure to have your lover swooning.

Here are some tips:

1. Don't overthink your email. Do what comes naturally, allowing yourself to tune into your sensual side. What are you thinking right now? What drives you crazy about your lover? What vivid images of the two of you intertwined take your breath away?

2. If you're stuck, think back to a shared sexual or sensual moment. What feelings are flooding your heart? What made the moment so memorable, so erotic? Use your words to re-create the moment's mood and meaning, showing how it still has a hold over your emotions—and lust quotient. Stress urgency: You're panting for your lover now, at this very must-get-naked-with-you moment.

3. Describe what you're feeling, thinking, and envisioning. Write about what you want to do, focusing on what turns your partner on. Describe your next rendezvous, your mounting desire, and how the moment can't come soon enough. Emphasize the physical, emotional, sexual, and spiritual elements of being with your lover, driving it home that you're deliciously distracted.

4. Remember, it's all in the details. Adjectives make or break your efforts. Be specific in your descriptions: What are you wearing (or not)? How are your senses coming alive? What does it feel like when . . . ?

TIME: 5+ minutes (depends on how quickly you write, your email's length, and if you are a perfectionist)

LUST-INDUCING LOCATION: anywhere that is not your place of work (unless, of course, you work from home)

MATERIALS: email access

PEAKING POTENTIAL: 1—you may feel a stirring in the loins, a sensation made into more effective foreplay with more passionate prose

139

Details like these make the picture you're painting come alive and can rev your lover's engine.

5. Read through your draft no more than a couple of times—too much revision can make it sound stale and overworked.

6. Come up with a creative subject line for the email that will make your lover stop whatever he or she is doing: "You have me wanting to . . ." "I was just thinking . . ." "I would love to . . ." "I'm touching my . . ." Use the first line of your text to complete the subject line.

7. Stoke your sweetie's fire without further adieu by clicking "Send."

Titillating Text Messaging

French (French kiss).
LOML (Love of My Life).
<3 (Heart).

Sending a text message (TM) has become all the rage, especially in the language of love. TMing is the perfect, convenient way to stay in touch throughout the day, keeping you charged 'til you can get all over each other. A 2008 Nielsen study found that 67 percent of unmarried texters who are dating or in a relationship use TMing to flirt.

Short and sweet, these messages instantly let you know that your honey is thinking of you. Romance goes from dull to daring with lines like, "Have you on my mind" to "WET4U." TMs also quickly and easily plant seeds for good times to come: "IWSN" (i.e., I want sex now), "2nite—no undies," "Can't wait 2CU," "SWAK" (i.e., sealed with a kiss), or even a simple "XOXO" (i.e., kisses and hugs). TMing is especially attractive to shy people who fear eye contact during any kind of sex communication, as well as for those of few words.

Adding to the excitement are cell phone vibrators, like the Toy Bluetooth vibe. With this device, partners wear a wireless, bullet vibe in or over their favorite hot spots. The vibrator is activated by texts sent to your phone. Lovers can experience solo sex simultaneously while sending each other scorching messages.

RULES OF ENGAGEMENT

The key to text messaging is knowing how to use it appropriately, known as "textiquette." *Don't* send a TM if:

➜ Your lover is at a business meeting. They're probably dying to hear from you, but there's a time and place to be hot and bothered.

➜ The respondent will have trouble understanding it. You have few words to work with. Don't waste them by being overly cryptic. Think short, sweet, and succinct. The aforementioned Nielsen survey found that 84 percent of texters think that TMs can be misunderstood by a date or suitor. People often need to ask for a second opinion of a message's meaning.

➜ You're delivering bad news about your sex life. No one deserves a "Ur bad n bed" text.

➜ You don't mean what you say and are simply being a tease.

➜ You're going to get bent out of shape if your love interest can't TM you back right away.

➜ It's the only way you plan to acknowledge a special day like Valentine's Day or your partner's birthday. You need to do more than just send a text!

The last point may surprise you. But a 2009 survey commissioned by AT&T Mobility and Consumer Markets involving more than a thousand eighteen- to fifty-five-year-olds found that 36 percent of texters were planning to send a text or picture message to celebrate Valentine's Day. If you ask me, these people are asking for trouble. Case in point: I once waited all day for my then-long-distance boyfriend to acknowledge Valentine's Day. When he finally did, it was with a simple "Happy V-day" text. My response: "I don't think you could've found a colder way to have said that." Now, I'm not somebody who makes a big deal out of Valentine's Day, but I was peeved by what I considered a lack of thoughtfulness—to the point that I had trouble appreciating the beautiful drawing he'd sketched for me to celebrate the holiday the following weekend. Call me old-fashioned, but I believe that texting can be used as an easy way out when it comes to sensual efforts. My advice: Don't rely on TMing to express your feelings—it's a fun addition to amore, but can't substitute for the real deal. Others agree: The AT&T study also found that TMing was an addition to other V-Day efforts: 67 percent planned to send an old-fashioned card, too.

1. Select your cell phone's camera option, and take a snapshot of your luscious self—the curve of your neck, your abs, your inner thigh.
2. Send the picture to your lover with the message: "Name This Curve."
3. Have fun going back and forth, getting racier if you dare, and adding flirtatious text to your steamy picture. Remember: Less is sometimes more, so a photograph of your bosom in your laciest lingerie could push your partner over the edge.

Note: When taking pictures, it's wise to leave out any identifying features like your face, tattoos, or birthmarks in case other people end up seeing the photos (e.g., if somebody finds your lover's lost mobile phone). Also, double-check that the picture is going to the intended recipient—and not to your mom or dad—before pressing "Send."

Intimate Instant Messages

Messager programs allow you and your sexy sidekick to send notes over the Internet, known as instant messages or IMs. Most IM programs enable you to communicate in a chat room or have a private discussion, share favorite web

TIME: 5 seconds

LUST-INDUCING LOCATION: body part of your choice

MATERIALS: camera phone

PEAKING POTENTIAL: 2—taking pictures of your sexiest features can easily get you aroused. If you then decide to take matters into your own hands, you may reach a 5 on the pleasure scale.

links, send videos, look at images stored on someone else's computer, play sounds, share files, and send IMs to a cell phone. Some, as we'll cover in the next section, also use a digital computer camera.

Like erotic emails and TMs, IMs provide people with freedom and instant gratification for sex communi-cation. IMing can be fast and flirty, emboldening you to express your sexual desires and fantasies. For many, masturbating goes hand-in-hand (pun intended) with this kind of real-time teasing. Almost one in three respondents in the 2008 UK Sex Report said they pleasured themselves while chatting on the Internet.

Some people, especially those in long-distance relationships, enjoy strategizing their IM seductions, like Tanjali: "In the beginning of my relation-ship, we lived in different cities so we relied a lot on instant messaging where we had erotic conversations in addition to sending one another dirty text messages and emails. Still, though, I think the sexiest thing was when I bought a new pair of tiny panties, wore them all day, and then mailed them to him without telling him what I was mailing. It made our next IM session even better."

RULES OF ENGAGEMENT

IMing is simple and allows you to practice all the erotic talk you've learned in this book. In setting up your IM experience, do the following:

→ Download an IM program (e.g., AOL's AIM or Yahoo's Messenger).
→ Read over your IM program's guidelines and regulations, which are often found in the Frequently Asked Questions section of the site. A few aren't down with dirty talk.
→ Don't send IMs to somebody at work unless you've been given the green light to do so. Only send an IM after you're positive that the recipient is at his or her desk; you don't want anyone intruding on your intimate space.
→ If the response you're drafting is lengthy, shoot a quick note back right away—something like: "Am sucking my tongue & working on a response, baby. . . ." That way, your special other won't feel blown off.
→ Turn your IM program off when you're not at your computer. Otherwise, your partner might attempt contact, believing you're online, and feel ignored.

1. Tell your lover ahead of time that the goal of this "sexercise" is to pretend that you don't know each other—you want to pick each other up for an online affair.

2. Set a sultry atmosphere by dimming the lights, playing sexy music, burning home fragrance oil, or whatever puts you in the mood. Make sure you're comfortable in your chair, sitting on a cushion, or propped against pillows on the bed.

3. Open your IM window and adjust the size of the dialog box, font type, font size, and color, with each reflecting the mood that you're after.

4. Begin your seduction: "My wife is in the other room. Wanna play?" "You're in luck. I'm alone and I just got out of the shower. I'm naked. Want a peek?"

5. Just like with offline sex, you want to warm up with foreplay. Work to arouse each other with professions of love and affection ("With you, my whole world has been transformed"), cheap thrills ("I can't wait to hear my cock slipping into your pussy"), or passionate provocation ("I'm hypnotized by the thought of watching you lick your lips before you go down on me").

6. No matter how far you choose to take things, aim for a sensory-rich experience—one inviting vivid pictures and describing your wanton desires with as much color and detail possible.

TIME: how much time do you have?

LUST-INDUCING LOCATION: any private space where you have Internet access

MATERIALS: computer with Internet access

PEAKING POTENTIAL: 3 if just IMing; 4 if masturbating while IMing

From Simple to Sophisticated: Sin-tillating Cybersex

While IMing is one way to turn up the heat, we've just scratched the surface. In submerging yourselves into cybersex, you can simulate sex by:

→ Smiling for the camera: Attach a digital webcam to the computer or use a computer's built-in webcam for whatever you fancy.

→ Meeting your lover or others in Internet chat rooms, such as IRC, or online virtual worlds, like Second Life, which are computer-based, imitation environments.

→ Adding your verbal allure with a voice chat system, such as Skype, that allows you to talk over the Internet free of charge.

→ Plugging in an audio-controlled device. Vibrators that work with a phone, microphone, television, or computer, such as Talk 2Me, turn sounds entering the transmitter's built-in microphone into stimulating vibrations.

Cybersex can have lovers pounding more than just the keyboard, getting lost in some serious voyeurism and exhibitionism. Commercial webcam sites offer observers the opportunity to watch others pleasuring themselves on camera. Public or private, these online trysts allow you to do more than spy by toying with Internet-enabled sex toys.

Teledildonics, a.k.a. cyberdildonics, involves the notion of telepresence. This is the experience of being "present" in real time within an online scenario, no matter where you actually are in reality. Such virtual sex is the closest thing to "real" sex since it utilizes sex toys, such as a vibrating faux penis or vagina, that are controlled by your computer over the Internet. Simply download the sex toy's software, plug the gadget into your computer, and voila: You and your lover can control one another's toys remotely online!

Cybersex enthusiasts are high on computer sex because it:

→ Allows for pleasure and sexual self-expression.
→ Provides opportunities to explore new "kinks," including sex acts and fetishes that a person wouldn't or couldn't experiment with in real life.
→ Builds confidence that helps with the real thing, including in-the-bedroom erotic talk.
→ Increases eroticism in existing intimate relationships, encouraging partners to explore sexual fantasies and role-playing.
→ Enables couples in long-distance relationships to feel connected.
→ Exercises exhibitionist tendencies when couples perform on camera for others to enjoy.
→ Liberates people who feel sexually inhibited to seek satisfaction.
→ Fuels ideas for sex scenes that can be acted out in real life.

There's also a polyamorous component to cybersex that appeals to some lovers. Encounters can involve more than two people having sex remotely via a computer network by sending "sexplicit" messages to the group, describing and responding to their activities. Alternatively, couples may enjoy drafting a sex script with a group of online participants while privately acting out sexually explicit passages at home. By having anonymity, participants can take on personas, owning the fantasy element, including trying a different gender or sexual orientation, with pleasure paramount.

Given there's no risk of getting pregnant or contracting a sexually transmitted infection, some argue that cybersex is safer than real sex. That is, as long as you don't give out your personal information to strangers.

One thing to be concerned about, for those using a webcam, is being recognized. It may be one chance in a million, but it's a chance worth considering given the repercussions of being spotted by your boss, spouse, or neighbor.

RULES OF ENGAGEMENT

Whether cybersexual on your own or as part of a couple, stick to the following guidelines:

→ Maintain a playful attitude. This is about having a good time!
→ Send your imagination into overdrive.
→ Suspend your disbelief. Don't get hung up on something feeling untrue. You've entered a fantasy world!
→ Guarantee yourself no interruptions.
→ Discuss virtual sex with your partner, setting rules that satisfy you both (e.g., what constitutes cheating online). Clarify boundaries up front.
→ Take your time. Build anticipation, raising the temperature through your words, thoughts, and movements.
→ Don't be shy about masturbating. You are, after all, simulating sexual behaviors.

And remember these don'ts—this advice may seem obvious, but it's worth considering if your cybersession is going to be all it can be:

→ Don't direct others on how to use cameras.
→ Don't be a creep.
→ Don't harass others.

Break any of these rules and you'll get kicked out of a community forum. Also avoid having cybersex in a public place, lest you get kicked out of that locale or worse, violate indececy laws. Finally, ask your e-flirt's age, since cybering with someone who's underage is illegal. Know, though, that it's very hard to confirm someone's age when your only contact is online.

Given there's no risk of getting pregnant

or contracting a sexually transmitted infection, some argue that cyber sex is safer then real sex.

Keep your online erotic talk efforts safe by following this advice:

1. Keep your personal ID private. Don't give it out to anybody you don't know.
2. Never agree to meet a stranger offline.
3. Never send pictures of yourself to a stranger.
4. Don't fill out a profile that asks for your private information.
5. Ask for a statement from your online playmate confirming that he or she is of adult age. Print the statement and keep it in a safe place.

Let cyberspace capture the rapture. Using your digital camera, put on an online strip show for each other by giving "Simon Says" a tantalizing twist.

1. For computers without a built-in camera, attach, install, and test a webcam.

2. Adjust the lighting in the room. You don't want any bright lights behind you. While a very dim room may be sensual for you, such lighting can make it hard to linger over every arousing detail (unless you want to obscure certain flaws or feel more comfortable performing in low light).

3. Make sure you look hot, if not dazzling.

4. Set aside uninterrupted private time and position yourself so that the camera captures all of you at a relatively close distance.

5. Choose who gets to be "Simon" first. That person starts by saying something like, "Simon says to unbutton your shirt."

6. If you're the one being told to do something, don't forget the erotic talk! Play up your part with comments: "Do you like that?" "Do you want a piece of this?" "Can I do anything else for you?" "Ooo, being bad feels so good!"

You could also play strip poker online and expose your exhibitionist impulses. Instead of playing for cash, you play for clothes, with an article of clothing lost for the one who loses a hand. Keep it simple if you're hot to see someone naked sooner rather than later. Also, decide beforehand what each article of clothing is worth: Is a sock worth one bet or two? How much for undergarments? You might decide that players can buy back articles of clothing— only to lose them again.

TIME: 20+ minutes (after installing and testing your webcam)

LUST-INDUCING LOCATION: in front of your digital camera

MATERIALS: web camera, computer with Internet connection

PEAKING POTENTIAL: 4, unless you masturbate—then it's 5

1. Install the device of your choice to a computer with an Internet connection, using a Windows operating system.

2. Fire up an audio component (e.g., Yahoo! Messenger). For those going all out, hook up your webcam.

TIME: 10 minutes for a quickie; 20+ minutes for a full-out sex session

LUST-INDUCING LOCATION: anywhere within 100 feet of your computer

MATERIALS: a penis masturbation sleeve called the Interactive Fleshlight (or other sex toy); a wireless vibrator called a Sinulator (plus its transmitter, receiver, and Rabbit vibrator); computer with Windows; audio component

PEAKING POTENTIAL: 5—Assuming you are comfortable with the set-up and toys

3. For your sci-fi-turned-reality sexual experience, go to Sinulator.com, name your sex toy, and make sure that whoever you're playing with knows the name of the toy you're allowing them to control.

4. The lover using the "Sinulator Cockpit" control panel should have a loose game plan as far as experimenting with different speeds and maneuvers. Begin pleasuring the partner who is using the Rabbit vibrator. (This is possible because the signals are sent through radio waves from your computer to the receiver to the sex toy.)

5. If you are using the vibrator on yourself, ask your lover to change the speed or rotation according to your wishes.

6. If you have the Interactive Fleshlight, you can slip this sleeve-style transmitter over a penis or dildo and start pleasuring yourself with it. The speed and thrust of your action will

be transmitted into vibrations that cause a pulse on the other end. So as you're thrusting, your partner's vagina or anus is being penetrated in response to your actions.

7. While lovers can get off on the action, especially if they're watching each other over a webcam, the sound component is what makes these moments red hot. Let loose and moan, squeal, or purr like mad. Share your every thought, from the pure ("You have me wanting nothing else") to the profane ("I'm so fucking hard thinking about spreading your cheeks and ramming you"). Putting it out there is critical if you're not using a webcam. Describe what's going on in lurid detail and make your thoughts and needs explicit, or your lover will be left guessing and you may be left unsatisfied.

Let loose and moan, squeal, or purr like mad.

Phenomenal Phone Sex

"You caught me just as I was getting out of the shower." "I'm lounging around in the brand new lingerie I bought today." "I just got off thinking about you."

Phone sex can catapult lovers into a sexual frenzy. It allows you to take risks and get dirtier than you might otherwise during face-to-face erotic talk. For couples separated by distance, phone sex can be fundamental to keeping the passion alive, as Alex knows well: "My long distance boyfriend and I have phone sex about once a week. It starts with mentioning how much I loved the last time we had sex, and then turns into me describing visions of how we are touching each other. We exchange ideas of what we want to do to each other. As the story builds, we both start touching ourselves and then try to cum together."

Phone sex, or "tele-fooling," is a vital form of communication for couples who are:

➜ Forced to be apart (e.g., due to military service or business travel)
➜ Hoping to eroticize their love life
➜ Dealing with a disability that prevents them from having other forms of sex
➜ Seeking safe ways to act out fantasies while staying monogamous
➜ Looking for a form of foreplay before they actually get together (e.g., when stuck at the office or in rush hour traffic)

No matter what your situation, this kind of tech sex boils down to your ability to be an erotic storyteller. It can entail:

➜ Telling each other what to do and acting on the suggestions
➜ Confessing sexual secrets and feelings
➜ Describing, in sensuous detail, how you're playing with yourself
➜ Listening to your partner masturbate

Phone sex can be romantic, nasty, or anything in-between, as Emiliana enjoys: "I love to hear the romantic, the dirty, the sweet, the sensual, the sexy. But it is also nice to be able to tell your lover what you like, your fantasies. It's equally nice to just talk about what you have done together and, before you know it, you are having phone sex, which is fun. Masturbating while you are talking on the phone is great, too. This helps in the bedroom, when you are actually having intercourse. I have to feel open to saying what I want when in person, and my lovers seem to love it, too. Phone sex helps me to do that."

Living together or continents apart, many lovers get off from satellite sex. A 2008 U.K. sex report found that 48 percent of women in Britain enjoy phone sex, and 50 percent of women and 44 percent of men who admit to liking dirty talk say they are likely to indulge in phone sex. Another survey by Internet phone company Vonage Canada found that 36 percent of Canadians have intimate phone conversations with a close "friend" or partner. The percentage jumped to 48 percent for those ages eighteen to thirty-four.

The interest is clearly there. But it can be intimidating to let loose your inner "slut" and kick things up a notch if you're worried about what to say. Remember: Phone sex should be a team effort, and shy lovers need to support each other until the process feels natural and takes on its own rhythm. If one partner is more confident about expressing sexually rapacious thoughts and suggestions, he or she should take the lead. But both lovers should approach phone sex as a game that's all about play and exploration.

If you're interested in giving phone sex a whirl, you and your partner may want to brainstorm scenarios that have erotic potential. All sorts of fictional situations can free you up and add to the fun. Think about these opening lines:

➜ "Operator, I need some assistance."
➜ "Oh, sorry—wrong number. Or maybe not, since I really like the sound of your voice."
➜ "Are you sure you have to go? Because I was just thinking that the next time I see you, I'm going to . . . "
➜ "I'm calling to inform you that you just won our grand prize drawing! Out of over 10,000 applications, your name was selected for the top prize— taking my virginity. If you can stay on the line, we need to figure out how you'd like to claim your prize."
➜ "Your voice makes me want to . . . "

RULES OF ENGAGEMENT

➜ Talk about what does and doesn't fly for both of you. For example, some people are not down with the idea of taking on a character; they want their lover to lust after them for who they are.

ANOTHER FORM OF PHONE SEX involves the commercial transaction between a paying customer and a paid sex worker, a.k.a. erotic actor, adult phone entertainer, or audio erotic performer. These phone sex professionals tap their talents as far as voice, acting, and role-playing in responding to a customer's requests. Scenarios may include a sex worker pretending to be masturbating, engaging in a particular type of sexual behavior, or fulfilling a customer's fetish fantasy. Calling this kind of hotline is a safe forum to "experience" taboo behaviors and can help people who are sexually inhibited, limited in their ability to physically perform, or who fear opening up to their committed partner about their desires. For example, some people have partners who will not partake in certain activities, so they seek gratification through commercial phone sex.

→ Consider using a landline if you need guaranteed privacy to feel relaxed. Cell and cordless phones are not always private.
→ Don't go to extremes—you're not going to confessional.

Usually, I discourage the use of clichés, but the oft-heard "What are you wearing?" can be a helpful ice-breaker that leads down other paths: "What would you like me to be wearing?" or "Actually, nothing. I was just about to slip into those lacy, red crotchless panties you love." Other ways to jumpstart the action include the following:

→ Start by leaving each other short, sexy voice mail messages: "I was just thinking about that time I woke up to your warm, wet lips wrapped around my cock, and how I made you cum so hard when I returned the favor." Doing so is like dropping a hot hint for sugar-sweet sexual liaisons to come, both on and off the line.

- Have fun using different voices, accents, tones, or roles to breathe new life into your aural art. Being able to blame a fictional persona for what came out of your mouth is what helps many people get naughty and tread new territory. For example, by pretending to be a French mistress, some women may feel emboldened to be a sultry vixen—even if that's not their personality. No matter what alter ego you choose, run with it and see where it takes you!
- Call your partner when you know you'll get his or her voice mail and record a sexy story after the tone. Continue the story until you're cut off at the hottest part. You can bet that your partner will call you back, begging to hear how the story ends.
- Describe something sexy you just did (or want to do): "I've just been trying on my new thong and garter!" or "I was thinking of you as I lathered my entire body during a long, steamy shower."
- Record erotic stories and play them back while you and your lover are on the phone and masturbating simultaneously. Let your breathing and sultry sounds add to the storyline.
- Buy a *Mad Libs* book and fill in the blanks with your sleaziest suggestions for verbs, adjectives, and nouns, composing your very own dirty magazine.
- Use a voice changer or software, such as AV Voice Changer Software Diamond edition, to transform your voice from male to female or vice versa, or make it sound robotic. This can add a humor or heighten the arousal because suddenly it's as if you're having phone sex with a total stranger.

Instead of calling your lover out of the blue, you may prefer to set up phone sex dates with a general plan in place. This gives both of you time to think about what you're going to say and how much you want to get into your role. Over time, however, you'll develop the confidence to have spontaneous phone sex, where both of you can corrupt each other without missing a beat.

Erotic Talk Action Plan: Putting Phone Sex Operators to Shame

We're about to explore three different exercises for your pleasure:

1. Erotically Charged Cliffhanger
2. Sinfully Sexy Storytelling
3. Playing with Myself

With each of these, consider . . .

What your lover likes. Craft your game plan accordingly, relying on what you know about your partner's body: "I'm brushing my soft lips across the back of your neck, breathing in the scent of you. You're giggling from light tickles of my warm breath on your nape before I start to work my way across your shoulder with gentle kisses, slowly reaching around to squeeze your pink, perky nipple with one hand, the other one going south to play with your. . ."

Rehearsing. Think about what you'll say, but keep things loose since your storyline can change at any moment, especially when your lover can direct the show by asking for more stroking, more humping, more nibbling.

Making sure that you have a clear phone connection. I once thought to tease a partner by calling him after an at-home workout. He picked up and, breathing heavily, I managed, "I am having so much fun with myself right now. Wish you were here." His reaction: "Huh?" I repeated myself, to which he again replied, "Huh?" Turns out we both had poor cell phone reception, ruining what could've been a kittenish come on.

Being articulate. Make sure that your lover can understand you. Seems obvious, but you don't want to be too quiet or mumble. If you're taking the time to choose your words carefully, you want to know that your lover understands every utterance.

Setting the mood. It can be hard to deliver a sultry performance when the TV is blaring in the background, a pot of water is boiling on the stove, or you're surrounded by unpaid bills. Adjust your environment to match the mood you're trying to create on the phone. For example, pour yourself a glass of wine and light candles.

Wearing what makes you feel sexy. Part of setting the mood is making sure you're comfortable, and that might mean stripping down to your birthday suit. (If you decide to play in the buff, make sure the room is warm enough. Teeth chattering isn't sexy.) If you don't feel the need to change your clothes, that's fine, but don't tell your lover that you're still in your sweats. When asked, describe your fantasy outfit (or his or hers) instead.

Teasing your body. You may not want to masturbate right away, but prepare your body and get yourself mentally psyched for what's coming (you, hopefully). Get comfortable, caress your skin, or gently touch your erogenous zones to awaken them. It usually helps to close your eyes and imagine that your lover is right beside you.

Calling with uninterrupted time. Phone sex can involve quickies, but serious sexual sessions are best when you're not worried about eavesdroppers or being interrupted. Do what's necessary to ensure your privacy.

Making the most out of pauses. While you don't want a silent stretch to last too long, your ability to skillfully use pauses can drive your lover mad, making him or her beg for more. You want the silences to last a second or two, but no longer than that, for fear that your lover will think the line has gone dead. Nothing can kill the moment like, "Are you there?"

Plan for a time when you know that your lover will be unable to answer his or her phone (e.g., working out at the gym or on an airplane).

TIME: 2 minutes (or as long as your lover's voice mail lasts)

LUST-INDUCING LOCATION: anywhere you don't have to lower your voice and where your amatory efforts won't offend those around you

MATERIALS: if you're not good with memorization or thinking off the top of your head, have your script handy

PEAKING POTENTIAL: 3—you will need to contain yourself 'til you can find some release

Before dialing your lover, think of things that will have you both burning with desire until you meet in person. Launching pad lines can include:

→ "I was just thinking that I love it when you put your _____ in my _____."
→ "I'm so horny right now, and I wish I was sliding my tongue all over your hot clit."
→ "I'm having visions of that time you had me bend over and. . . ."

Ring your partner, and with a cool confidence, unmask your orgasmic thoughts.

Ideally, you want the voice mail to cut you off right before you reach the "climax" of your mini-work. (Note: This may require a trial run. A week before, call your lover's voicemail, armed with a stopwatch, and babble about your day as you time how long you've got before getting cut off.)

Reading erotic stories to your lover may be one way to take the pressure off your own writing skills while still taking things to another level with your partner. Plus, reading from an existing work can supply you with new ideas for when you go back to compose original material. So curl up with a raunchy read as you learn to be a supernatural sex power with your lover hanging on your every word.

Delivery is everything, so read over what you're going to say, practicing segments in a rich, deep, husky voice and paying attention to points in the plot that benefit from a pause before proceeding. Consider where your voice can add more color to the story and really lift it off the page and bring it to life. You want your lover to be unable to concentrate on anything other than what's coming out of your mouth.

And if you get swept away, you can always pick up where you left off the next time you get together. Ashton swears by it: "Dear Penthouse, I never thought this would happen to me. We had a date night where I set up a room with two comfy chairs facing each other. I put some electronic tango jazz on low volume, and then on another stereo I put on erotic recordings of sex stories. I put porn movies on the TV, muted, and over all that we read sex stories from Penthouse Letters. Sometimes we read them out loud or talked about what we were reading. After a half an hour and some wine, we were both pretty juiced. That went more than well."

TIME: 25 minutes (depending on the length of your story and your stylistic efforts)

LUST-INDUCING LOCATION: preferably in your bed or on the couch

MATERIALS: erotic literature, such as Nancy Friday novels or *Penthouse Forum*

PEAKING POTENTIAL: 3.5—higher with self-pleasuring

The aim of this exercise is to create an erotic mental picture for your lover that features you playing with yourself. Sound effects are like special effects—they heighten the experience—so don't be afraid to pant, moan, groan, purr,

TIME: 25 minutes

LUST-INDUCING LOCATION: your bedroom

MATERIALS: any notes you need to stay on your task of tempting

PEAKING POTENTIAL: 4.5—it may be hard to stay focused on pleasuring yourself while trying to drive your audience wild

and whisper to prompt your lover to react. Other than that, you can take any number of directions:

→ Describe what you're wearing (even if it's fantasized), letting your lover know how it feels to slip off every piece of clothing.

→ Let your lover know what you're doing to yourself, detail by detail: "I'm spreading the lips of my soaking wet slit."

→ Explain every phase of your arousal: "I'm stroking myself, faster and faster, feeling like I'm about to explode when I think about you riding me."

→ Alternatively, pretend that your partner is there with you: "Your fingers are crawling up my short skirt, searching for my underwear—only to find that I'm not wearing any," or "I can feel your stubble rubbing against my inner thigh."

→ Be affectionate when it fits the bill: "I wish I could feel your warmth lying next to me."

If you're on the listening end, respond to what's being described by doing any of the following:

→ React to the description. For example, moan when your lover says, "I'm pinching my nipples."

→ Tell your lover how much you are getting off from his or her most precious parts: "You're putting your fingers in your mouth. Now put those slippery wet digits between your legs. I want to see those fingers sliding into your lovely dripping cunt."

→ Dish out the details of your sexual response: "I'm getting harder and harder, my sac pulsating, my cock flushed, my tip glistening from what's about to come."

→ Make requests: "I want you to rub my tits as you_____." or "Say that again."

Know that you don't have to make your phone sex sessions terribly long. You can start a scenario and then your lover can react with a comeback of his or her own, building your story together. Or you can go for a quickie, like the example on the next page, reading it as though it were poetry.

I'm in my dark green rayon top,

The one with the buttons I accidentally never button up.

Leaning over you,

Slightly pressing,

Knowing your eyes are eagerly undressing

This little vixen I've become.

A slow and sensual lap dance

Mission accomplished—mmm—wet pants

I'm getting off on your moans and deep breaths.

Do you like that I'm being a tad too fresh?

Chapter 5 Check-In

This chapter introduced you to the many ways you and your lover can satisfy each other with tech sex. In evaluating how things went, ask yourself the following:

→ What specific activities led to abundant arousal? Which ones did nothing for one or both of you?

→ Which forms of tech sex—emails, TMs, IMs, cybersex, or phone sex—have the potential to turn you on, even if they didn't work as hoped for the first go-around? Could you change the storyline, try role-playing, buy enhancements to take advantage of the technology?

→ Do you need to tweak the rules of engagement to improve results?

→ What was it about these erotic talk expeditions that excited you and suggests they're worth trying again?

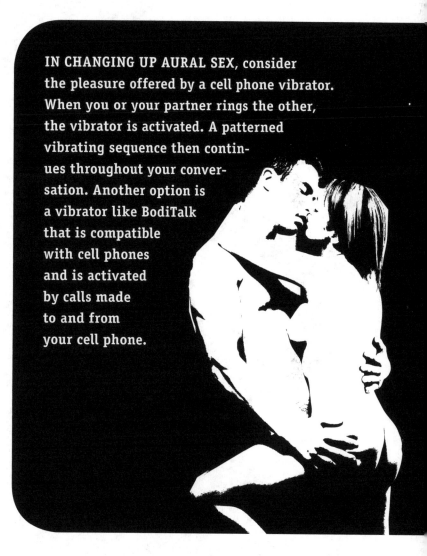

IN CHANGING UP AURAL SEX, consider the pleasure offered by a cell phone vibrator. When you or your partner rings the other, the vibrator is activated. A patterned vibrating sequence then continues throughout your conversation. Another option is a vibrator like BodiTalk that is compatible with cell phones and is activated by calls made to and from your cell phone.

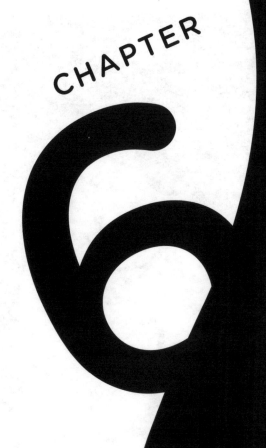

CHAPTER

6

Sexplorations:
Where Will Your Tongue Take You?

IN CHAPTER 6, YOU'LL LEARN HOW TO:

- ❦ Kick up your capacity for fantasy.

- ❦ Master rock-star sex via role-playing.

- ❦ Fuel your passion with endless ideas for years to come.

" Group sex,
same sex,
threesomes, swinging,
sex with the other's sibling. . . . You name it, we've
probably fantasized about it and anything goes
when it comes to sharing. We've been together
since junior high school, and part of keeping our
sex life hot involves pushing the envelope with
what gets us going and what we might want
to try. Sometimes we'll build the fantasy
together, trying to up each other with the
shock value. The more taboo the better
as far as feeling closer to each other in
having such a safe space for sharing
fantasies as with no one else. "

AS MIKE'S COMMENTS illustrate, lovers get a huge thrill out of sexual fantasies, and everyone, whether they admit or realize it, has the ability to fantasize. I say this as someone who once thought otherwise. I was in graduate school, taking a sexual behaviors course, when the class discussion turned to phantasms (those figments of your imagination). My confession was that I'd never had a sexual fantasy. Sure, we were studying others' fantasies—people who wanted to have sex with elderly people (gerontophilia), people who would visit a dominatrix to act out their diaper fetish, people who had a thing for latex. Never one to let myself sit around and have sexy thoughts, let alone desire such, I admired others' abilities to let their imaginations run wild.

My professor didn't believe I'd never had a sexual fantasy. Trying not to embarrass me, he delicately asked if I'd ever had a crush on somebody. "Most definitely!" I replied. He then asked if I ever daydreamed about kissing that somebody. I said yes to that, too. He broke into a smile and said, "Well, you see then, you have had a sexual fantasy!"

Whether deliberate or unexpected, we humans have an enormous capacity to craft and run with erotic mental imagery, sending sexual excitement into overdrive. Even a flash thought, from the mild to the exotic, can launch you into an erotic orbit.

Solo or together, lovers use these thoughts, these passports to pleasure, to increase sexual feelings and explore their sexual selves. This type of heady sex, whether a fleeting image or an elaborate screenplay, can be a revelation to lovers as they discover the "phantastic" side of their eroticism. How much you fantasize and what you find sexy varies from person to person. This can change over time and with certain circumstances (talk to any lusty preggie in her orgasmic prime, and you'll know what I mean).

Perhaps the best thing is that anything goes when it comes to your personal fantasies. There are no rules in this mindblowing, make-me-moan microcosm of yours. You're totally in charge. You only have to pleasure yourself. You can have the best sex imaginable with anyone, anywhere you want, whether that's Scarlett Johansson in the back of your beat up VW van or Johnny Depp on the red carpet in front of the paparazzi. Nobody will to turn you down; nobody will put cuffs on you (unless that's part of your plot). You can concoct anything you want, and who's going to be the wiser—and sexier—for it? You.

People have all sorts of fantasies, from the loving to the lurid—and those fantasies can involve any of the erotic talk themes we've explored. Romantic could be making love for the first time, while sensual might be taking a double

dip in the Playboy mansion swimming pool with the Miss July and August centerfolds. Or perhaps you get hard imagining that you're getting a golden shower from a stunning domme who's pinning you down with the heel of her four-inch stilettos (literally dirty).

What's radical for one person is conservative to the next, so don't worry your pretty little head over what's inside your mind. Wherever you fall on the spectrum of "tame" to "hardcore" of sexual fantasies, it is just right for you.

Being able to fantasize is a natural part of healthy sexuality. So let your fantasy play out in your head without editing your sexy thoughts, and invite their many benefits. Fantasy:

➜ Is sex when you find yourself alone.
➜ Eroticizes sex for greater sensations when you're using condoms or dental dams. (As I said in *The Hot Guide to Safer Sex*, if your mind is lost in a phantastic orgasm, protected sex is just as sweet.)

- Helps couples stay monogamous for the long haul.
- Can be done anytime, anywhere.
- Costs nothing.
- Can help you overcome sexual anxieties and boost your sexual self-esteem with visions of your worship-worthy performance.
- Feeds you (and your relationship) with new, fresh, and daring ideas.
- Can make you feel sexier, more attractive, powerful, adored, and desired.

- Is a fast, effective way to get aroused.
- Helps you *oh-oh*-orgasm.
- Can intensify your sexual experience and pleasuring.

Quiz: Unearthing Your Fantasies

From this point forward, we're going to explore your fantasies, figuring out which ones should be shared, acted out, or never breathed. In uncovering these natural aphrodisiacs, we're going to begin with a quiz to determine what's going on in your own wanton world. Circle all choices that apply.

1. **The following statement(s) describe my fantasies overall:**
   a. They involve a particular context/situation.
   b. The envisioned encounters evoke a lot of feelings.
   c. If I were to share them, they would be rich in description.
   d. They focus on specific sexual acts.
   e. They involve a lot of visual content.

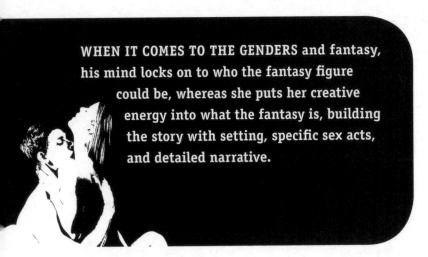

WHEN IT COMES TO THE GENDERS and fantasy, his mind locks on to who the fantasy figure could be, whereas she puts her creative energy into what the fantasy is, building the story with setting, specific sex acts, and detailed narrative.

f. They focus heavily on my sex object's genitals.

g. They're heavy on my fantasy partner's responses and physical appearance.

h. The storylines build slowly to explicit activity.

i. They involve affection.

j. They're passionate.

k. They're romantic.

l. They're sensual.

m. They focus on my (real or imagined) partner's physical or emotional characteristics.

n. They involve doing things that I would never do in real life.

2. **The people in my fantasies tend to be:**

   a. Current partner(s)

   b. Past partners

   c. Imaginary partner(s)

   d. People with whom I'm familiar

   e. An authority figure.

   f. Other: _____

   g. I don't tend to fantasize about people as much as _____

3. **The following describe(s) the power dynamics that are a theme in my fantasies:**

   a. I am dominant (in charge).

   b. I am forcing another against their will.

   c. I am the object of desire.

   d. I am the active partner. (I'm doing/guiding the action.)

   e. I am the passive partner. (I'm having the action done to me.)

   f. I'm irresistible and wanted.

   g. I'm chasing the object of my desire, successful in my sexual conquest.

   h. Other: _____

4. Rate the following sexual behaviors.

Fantasy Potential	"Turns me on."	"Makes me really hot."	"Turns me off."	"Disturbs me."
Sex with a stranger	O	O	O	O
Sex in a public place	O	O	O	O
People around me being naked	O	O	O	O
Being sexually victimized	O	O	O	O
Sacrilegious sex acts	O	O	O	O
Indecently exposing myself	O	O	O	O
Putting on a strip show	O	O	O	O
Masturbating in private	O	O	O	O
Masturbating in a public place	O	O	O	O
Joining the "Mile High Club" (sex in an airplane)	O	O	O	O
Elevator sex	O	O	O	O
Being promiscuous	O	O	O	O
Having sex with another couple	O	O	O	O
Watching men and women masturbate	O	O	O	O
Sex outside	O	O	O	O
Sex with a call girl/stripper	O	O	O	O
Double penetration	O	O	O	O
Dressing up in leather	O	O	O	O
Being videotaped	O	O	O	O
Dressing up in plastic or rubber	O	O	O	O
Cross-dressing	O	O	O	O
Same-sex scenarios	O	O	O	O

Fantasy Potential	"Turns me on."	"Makes me really hot."	"Turns me off."	"Disturbs me."
Heterosexual scenarios	O	O	O	O
Watching people have intercourse	O	O	O	O
Group sex	O	O	O	O
Forced sex	O	O	O	O
Threesomes	O	O	O	O
Erotic talk	O	O	O	O
Sex with an ex	O	O	O	O
Sado-masochism (S&M)	O	O	O	O
A specific fetish: _____	O	O	O	O
Using a particular sex toy: _____	O	O	O	O
Gender play	O	O	O	O
A specific sex act: _____	O	O	O	O
Reliving a previous sexual experience	O	O	O	O
Going to a sex club	O	O	O	O
Swinging	O	O	O	O
Circle jerk (male group masturbation)	O	O	O	O
Fisting	O	O	O	O
Quickie sex	O	O	O	O
Oral sex on a woman	O	O	O	O
Oral sex on a man	O	O	O	O
Sex in specific or different positions	O	O	O	O
Having sex in public with high risk of being seen/discovered	O	O	O	O

Time for true confessions: Have you fantasized about a number of these scenarios? Did you find yourself getting excited just eyeballing this list? Well, you're in good company. Lots of people fantasize about many of these behaviors. Many of these fantasies, however, are never acted upon. It's not that people are afraid to give them a go or fear they'll end up in jail; it's that preserving these acts as fantasies keeps them potent and taboo, always there for you when you want to get sexed up or relish sexual release.

Spike Your Sex Drive by Sharing Sexy Thoughts

Everyone's heard that our biggest sex organ is the brain, and it's true: Your orgasmic response is based in your brain more than in your genitals. With that in mind, lovers can play this instrument of desire by sharing their fantasies through erotic talk. It's only natural for lovers to want to disclose some of their pent-up passions. By revealing select top secret sex files, they turn up the heat and open the door to an entirely new world of sexual expression. Sharing naughty thoughts helps keep the action hot and the passion alive by stimulating the body's release of its own natural drugs, ones that nourish our basic drive for love and attachment.

As the brain engages in fantasy play, it becomes aroused, releasing chemicals that send more blood to

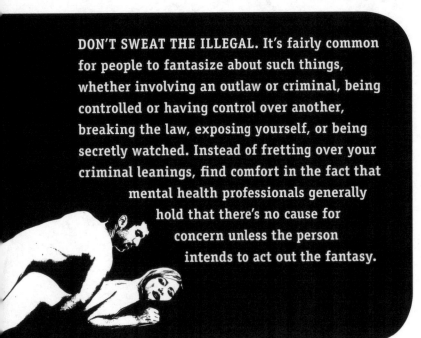

DON'T SWEAT THE ILLEGAL. It's fairly common for people to fantasize about such things, whether involving an outlaw or criminal, being controlled or having control over another, breaking the law, exposing yourself, or being secretly watched. Instead of fretting over your criminal leanings, find comfort in the fact that mental health professionals generally hold that there's no cause for concern unless the person intends to act out the fantasy.

your erogenous zones. Dopamine, in particular, is one of the chemicals that can motivate you and your partner to get better acquainted, driving your behavior until you feel nearly possessed. When dopamine levels in the brain increase, so does the level of testosterone, cranking up sexual desire in both men and women.

So how do you boost your supply of this natural upper? Anything new, edgy, or forbidden that has the power to excite and motivate increases dopamine levels, while anything routine lessens it. So unexplored sexual experiences elevate dopamine levels and trigger lust, which is why erotic talk, fantasies, and role-playing are your admission tickets to your own X-rated rendezvous.

By talking about and acting out fantasies, lovers renew their attraction and reinforce their lust for each other, as Jermaine knows: "Talking about and acting out our fantasies helps us both explore areas of our sexuality we might otherwise be afraid to explore. Talking about what we've been thinking in our heads—bringing fantasies from our private thoughts to the forefront of our relationship—is a way of slowly expanding and pushing limits. Doing it through sexy talk is what works for us, allowing us to safely say what we are sometimes embarrassed to share since the focus is on getting sexed up through erotic talk."

RULES OF ENGAGEMENT

Bringing your sexual phantasms to light with another person can feel scary at first. It's easy to feel shy, unsure, or apprehensive if you're worried about embarrassing yourself or shocking your partner. The benefits are worth the risk, though, as long as there's enough trust to bring someone into your sexual confidence. To invite sharing, make lovers feel safe, supported, and understood with the following tactics:

➡ Be open-minded. Consider a fantasy's potential for improving your sex life and making you feel closer as a couple.

➡ Timing is everything. Resist blurting out fantasies at inappropriate times (e.g., telling her you start to pant at the thought of virgin sex as you're driving past a high school field hockey practice).

→ Be patient with each other. It may take a while for someone who feels shy and tongue-tied to fully express a thought or to react to what's being shared. Be a caring listener and ask for something to be clarified or repeated if necessary.

→ Agree that saying something doesn't necessarily mean that you want to do it. Never put pressure on a partner to act out a fantasy. Don't be afraid, however, to mention which fantasies have the potential for role-play.

→ Don't force the other person to share something they'd rather keep private. If your lover withholds fantasies, it is not a sign that you're not emotionally close or that there's something wrong with the relationship. Everyone has a right to their private thoughts.

→ Don't ambush your partner. Like we covered in other erotic talk activities, don't take a "let's talk now" approach. Make a request to share, and then give them time to process if necessary.

→ If you don't like what you hear, don't punish your partner with criticism or negativity, or by withdrawing physically or emotionally. We're all unique and individual responses must be respected.

→ As with any type of erotic talk, keep it in moderation, as Carlos learned the hard way: "With my ex-wife, we were extremely successful playing out *all* fantasies verbally—to the point that we almost couldn't have sex unless we were discussing a fantasy or reliving a past sexual experience."

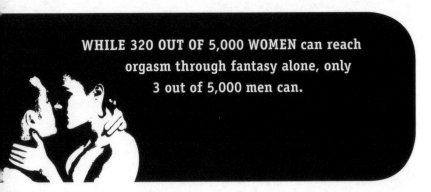

WHILE 320 OUT OF 5,000 WOMEN can reach orgasm through fantasy alone, only 3 out of 5,000 men can.

"Get naked" takes on a whole new meaning when it involves divulging your sexual nature at its deepest level. In this action plan, you'll strip down to your rawest and most ravenous selves and unfurl your sexual energy as you:

1. Decide what you want to share
2. Give thought to what your partner can handle
3. Let it all hang out—almost

Communicating about your fantasies and carnal curiosities should be thrilling and fun, and it will be as long as you're both comfortable and create a welcoming space in which to share. In freeing yourselves to describe and trade fantasies, you'll understand each other better and have a new realm for testing your sexual limits. With this powerful, sensual awakening, you may see yourself and your partner differently. This change can invite a new chapter in your relationship—one that's more playful, more daring, and includes more opportunities for sex, including

the "how tos" of making your honey horny and happy.

1. **Contemplate what and why you want to share.** Thanks to the quiz you took earlier, you have a better sense of what tickles your fancy. Now think about the items you want to share—as well as anything not covered in that exercise— and consider why each is worth

TIME: take your time

LUST-INDUCING LOCATION: a private place where you both feel comfortable

MATERIALS: none, although the quiz on pages 97–100 (without your answers filled in) might be helpful for bringing on action

PEAKING POTENTIAL: 3.5—this can be as exciting as you want it to be!

mentioning. Do you just want to get a few things off your chest? Or do you want to share every discovery about your seductive "dark" side? Do you see sharing as a type of foreplay? Are you hoping that some of what you share will turn into games or inspire role-playing? Weigh the pros and cons of sharing as a benefit to the relationship versus just for you: Does sharing that you fantasize about doing your fitness trainer doggie style serve any purpose beyond exciting you? What does your partner or your union stand to gain by knowing that? This is especially important to consider when it comes to fantasies that involve more risk, such as unveiling the fact that your fantasies hint at more bisexual urges than you've ever acted on, a tidbit that could rattle less open-minded lovers. Consider, too, that keeping certain fantasies all to yourself may be more

to your advantage when it comes to self-pleasuring—for example, if you're tired and feeling pressure to cum and know a particular thought sequence will get you to sweet slumber by way of a heavenly orgasm.

2. **Be realistic about what your relationship can handle.** Swapping fantasies treads on sexual territory that not every relationship can hack. You'll be making yourselves vulnerable and, as with trying different kinds of erotic talk, both of you must withhold judgment when revealing some of your deepest, most personal devilish desires. Be sensitive and empathetic when your partner opens up to you: "I know that that wasn't easy to share. Thanks for trusting me."

3. **Know what your lover can handle.** Some partners are perfectly cool with whatever and whoever comprises their lover's personal

storybook, but others aren't quite as tolerant. They may view a sexual fantasy as a type of emotional affair. They may feel jealous knowing that you want to bend over the desperate housewife next door or watch your roommate's legs spread wide during a housemate orgy. Don't waste your time attempting to share if your partner sees any fantasy that doesn't entail just the two of you as disturbing. If you're not sure what or how much your partner can handle, buy a book on fantasies as a nice surprise and ask if that can be your new bedtime reading. Or rent a movie featuring your fantasy to gauge your partner's reaction.

4. **Be savvy about how you share.**
Start your discussion by sharing tamer fantasies, as these tend to be easier both to articulate and digest. Just be sure to edit any details that may cause jealousy or trigger a misunderstanding. This is especially true of the people in

the scenes you describe because, as mentioned above, some lovers find it unacceptable to have anybody but themselves in the starring role. You don't want your lover to feel threatened by or less desirable because of your phantasms. Should this happen, reassure your lover that you are satisfied with the relationship and you don't actually plan to get off at the same bus stop for an anonymous tryst with that hottie you've been checking out on the commute home.

You can also comfort your lover with the fact that most people's fantasies involve others who aren't their partner. One study found that 87 percent of participants had fan-tasized about someone other than their current partner in the past two months. This kind of window-shopping is part of what enables lovers to remain faithful.

5. **Be sensitive in how you react.**
Throughout the conversation with your lover, respond to what is

shared, even if it's just saying something like "I'm really touched that you opened up about that." Silence can be hard to read in these situations and may cause distress. And as with any sex talks, don't ridicule your partner or make fun

of the fantasy he or she shares with you. Make sure that both of you are in the know when it comes to the different types of fantasies people have because normalizing them will make them less threatening. Common themes in fantasies include:

→ Forbidden fantasies, like affair sex, which heart-poundingly violate social norms and moral strictures. Going against what has been deemed "proper" sexual behavior has the power to arouse, especially if it involves an abuse of power (e.g., a high school teacher who insists that his innocent, young student stay late for extra attention or else).

→ Force fantasies. While illegal in real life, these center on a "victim" who is so irresistible that the other is overcome with desire and willing to do anything and everything to obtain the sex object. The aggressor gets off on being overpowering and sexually invincible.

FANTASIZING ABOUT the love affair between you and your partner can be some of the sexiest stuff to share. During pillow talk, tell a bedtime story, reminiscing about shared sexual moments that are highlights of your relationship, adding a slight twist if you feel so inspired. It will give you both a "sweet dreams" send-off.

→ Starring role fantasies, in which you might be a supermodel, celebrity, or musician. These are some of the easiest to admit.

→ Movie- or television-borne fantasies. Imagine having a romance like Ryan Gosling and Rachel McAdams in *The Notebook*, or re-creating the "this rose is for you" scene from *The Bachelor*, where the eligible bachelor selects the winning contestant who's been vying with the competition for true love.

Ask questions, in part to learn more details, but also to find ways to expand your realm of pleasuring: "Is that something you hope we'll do as a role-play?" or "Is that something you want to replicate?"

Entering into the conversation with a positive, eager attitude will have its pay-offs, as Max reports: "It's hard to share and hear fantasies, but definitely a good idea in the long run. Some topics feel threatening at first—for example, if you fantasize about a threesome. At first your partner might feel inadequate or threatened by that. But if you discuss it, you can talk about why you fantasize about it and it will likely become less threatening."

Rock Your World Role-Playing

Once you've both put your fantasies out there, it's time to turn your sex life into a pleasure playground. In this section of the book, your task is to determine what's intriguing enough to pursue together by using our suggestions, tips, and sample scenarios for transforming your imagining into reality. Remember that no matter the story you're building or the atmosphere you're trying to create, there must be a sense of safety for when exploring one's sexual alter egos and testing out new territory. Listen to what Wally had to say about the rape fantasy he used to act out with his ex-girlfriend: "She'd bring it up and [would] put on dressy clothes—like skirts, stockings, lingerie—and ask me to chase her around the house. Basically, she would act like she was trying to get away from me. It involved grabbing a hold of her, pushing her down over a chair, removing her underwear, and having sex with her. She'd squirm to 'act' like she didn't want it. I'd hold her and make it so she couldn't get away. Eventually, we'd work toward regular sex, since we usually did that on our power session, 'sex marathon' days. . . . I never objected to the rape fantasy. We had a fairly active sex life, did unusual things. I, though, never wanted to bring it up for fear of making her mad or upset. I didn't want to push it on her. I wanted her to want to do it, too. And I guess we had the safe space in which she felt we could do this."

RULES OF ENGAGEMENT

When you and your partner are ready to get into character, take a moment to agree on the following rules:

→ You can politely and unapologetically refuse a request: "While it's nice of you to take a chance by suggesting that, I don't think that it's something I'm willing to try."

→ Don't refuse a suggestion with a "never." That blanket response can shut down communication. And who knows? You might just change your mind one day.

→ If something doesn't sound quite right, suggest an alternative activity that's close to what's being requested but tweaked a bit to suit your tastes. For example, instead pretending to be picked up at a bar for casual stranger sex, maybe you'd rather pretend that you are old high school lovers who meet again after years and all too easily rekindle your romance.

→ Don't get upset if things don't go as expected. Roll with it, and look forward to a better experience the next time.

→ Don't see incompatibilities as defects. People have a number of likes and dislikes when it comes to sex. You're not always going to be on the same page, and that's okay. It's not an indicator that there's something wrong with either of you or with the relationship.

→ Check in with each other to process the role-play in terms of how things are going and how you feel, especially to assess if anything needs to be adjusted.

Your mission is to come up with a co-created role-play activity that will have both of you feeling scrumptiously sexual. In settling down to write your script, discuss the following questions for starters, explaining your expectations, the appeal of each, and any apprehensions, plus all of the details, to make sure that you're psychologically prepared for anything that could come up. When crafting your screenplay, stay erotically focused. Your lover will be intrigued to learn why you think a certain outfit is a must, what's important to say when, and what it is about every step in the plan that turns you on. The smart lover will take mental notes to incorporate into future sex sessions.

TIME: remember, time flies when you're having fun, so set aside at least an hour so you can take a leisurely approach

LUST-INDUCING LOCATION: your choice

MATERIALS: your choice

PEAKING POTENTIAL: depends on your fantasy

WHO IS IN THE FANTASY?
➜ Just the two of you
➜ Stranger(s)
➜ Old lover(s)
➜ Prostitute(s)
➜ Stripper(s)
➜ Dominatrix (dominatrices)
➜ Colleague(s)
➜ Classmate(s)
➜ Famous person (people)
➜ Friend(s)
➜ Character(s) (e.g., Cat Woman, James Bond)
➜ Other:_____

WHERE WILL THIS TAKE PLACE (REAL OR PRETEND)?

The Great Outdoors
➜ Woods
➜ Secluded picnic area
➜ Lake
➜ Ocean
➜ Field
➜ Waterfall
➜ Under moonlight
➜ City park
➜ Orchard
➜ Beach
➜ Playground
➜ Nudist retreat
➜ Dark alley

Geographically Speaking
➜ Foreign country
➜ Famous historical landmark
➜ Deserted island
➜ Lighthouse
➜ Space
➜ Paradise

Travel Plans
➜ Plane
➜ Train
➜ Motorcycle
➜ Car
➜ Hot air balloon
➜ Camping
➜ Ski lodge
➜ Motel
➜ Ship
➜ Boat
➜ Canoe
➜ Hotel
➜ Resort
➜ Bed and breakfast
➜ Restroom
➜ Carriage ride

Buildings
➜ Movie theater
➜ Library
➜ Sports club
➜ Performing arts theater
➜ School
➜ Museum
➜ Haunted house

- → Castle
- → Mansion
- → Room in your house
- → Barn

Other
- → Time travel
- → Old West
- → Hollywood movie set

- → Backstage at a concert
- → Amusement park
- → Elevator
- → Jacuzzi

WHAT TYPES OF ACTIVITIES ARE INVOLVED?
- → Erotic talk
- → Peep show
- → Strip club
- → Burlesque show
- → Spanking
- → Gender play
- → Certain positions
- → Fondling of genitals
- → Breast play
- → Sex toys
- → Strap-on and dildo
- → Fingering
- → Rimming (anal-oral contact)
- → Anal intercourse
- → Cunnilingus
- → Fellatio
- → Bondage
- → Sado-masochism (S&M)
- → Vaginal-penile intercourse
- → Other: _____

PRETENDING THAT YOU and your lover are meeting for the first time is one of the oldest tricks in the book, but it still works, as Hayden can tell you: "My [significant other] and I go to restaurants, bars, etc., and pretend we are different people. Sometimes it turns goofy, but sometimes we keep up the act all evening, only to end up in the sack together for a 'one-night stand.' "

To avoid becoming too much like plotless male-oriented porn (unless that's your wish), decide on how you'll launch things by setting the stage with a fantastical world. In this fantasy, how do you know each other or how did you meet? Now brainstorm the main points of your extraordinary adventure: the seduction, the suspense, the erotic dance, the conquest, the ultimate release.

To fill in your plotline, consider these questions:

→ Do you have fake names (if acting out characters)?
→ Is the scene set during a specific period in history (e.g., medieval era)?
→ Do you need props or supplies for set design (e.g., food, wigs, or furniture)?
→ What will you do to become your character (e.g., play up an accent, use the lingo of a certain period of time, or change your voice)? What do you know about the character's personal history or backstory? What makes this character alluring? What's not going to work for either of you in taking on this character's role?
→ What will you wear (e.g., do you want to rent costumes or can you assemble outfits from what you already own)?
→ Would it be fun to include sexual enhancers (e.g., lube or a feather boa) for spine-tingling reactions?
→ Have you agreed on a word or sign for stopping the action?
→ Is your privacy assured (e.g., housecleaning isn't going to knock on the door in the middle of your *Pretty Woman* reenactment)?
→ Is there something specific that you'd like to see happen during the scene for maximum arousal (e.g., "I'd love for you to pin my arms over my head as you take me")?

With some of the basic details sorted out (remember you should leave space for spontaneity and improvisation), go ahead and lose yourself in your character, tailoring the role to fit your personality. Step into the world of your shared fantasy and see where your words, gestures, and actions lead you—which will hopefully be to new realms of erotic thrills and sensual delights.

KEEP THE GAMES GOING by occasionally describing an erotic dream. These soulful, symbolic visions act as a good excuse for unveiling areas we're afraid to explore, inviting a deeper connection with ourselves and our lover. In showing us what's fun and why, these dreams provide us with even more stimulating ideas for a stronger relationship.

For lovers looking for ideas for crafting your fantasy, consider the following as starting points for your efforts.

The Phantasm: Next-Door Neighbor
The Setting: For months you've been checking out the next-door neighbor, drooling over this sexy thing's glistening skin and toned body stretched out by the backyard pool.

The Climax: Today, your favorite sunbather is soaking up the rays perfectly nude. And instead of merely watching sunscreen get applied, you decide that this may be the day to bring over a neighborly gift, like chocolate body paint, which may require a good washing in the pool after you've licked it all off.

The Phantasm: Yogis on Sabbatical
The Setting: You've escaped to a hot naked yoga retreat for some serious rest and relaxation. After working up a good sweat, you feel incredibly free, flexible,

and sensual as you settle into a cross-legged, seated position and close your eyes.

The Climax: You're surprised, but your interest is piqued, when you feel a silky blindfold being placed over your eyes. Your senses come alive with anticipation as you feel a chilled berry slowly making its way across your lips. You feel intoxicated by the faceless one's seductive scent, and catch your breath as you find yourself being gently straddled, your seductor's legs wrapping around your waist. As you breathe in harmony, you wonder when you'll get to look in the other's eyes.

The Phantasm: Cop and Speeder

The Setting: You've just been pulled over for speeding by a supersexy cop. You actually don't mind when the cop starts to rough you up a bit. In fact, you're a little disappointed when the cop goes back to the police car.

The Climax: The cop returns, telling you to lean against the car for more frisking—only this isn't your average frisk. Fingers are lingering on your palpitating hot spots this time, and you can't believe your luck as you feel the stimulating ripples of a butt plug enter you. The cop breathes in your ear. "I just called in for back up."

The Phantasm: Underage Prostitute and Customer

The Setting: You've solicited a sex worker for some serious sexual release. Only when she walks into your place, you're a bit surprised that your Lolita-like fantasy is about to come true.

The Climax: Even though you planned it, and even though you're paying for it, you can hardly believe it when your prostitute says, "I want to feel you inside me—again." With hips gripped, you enter again, using slow, steady strokes until, with one tight backside pressing harder against you, you go over the edge when you hear, "That's it, fuck me. I want it."

The Phantasm: French Film Director and Actor

The Setting: You have the leading role in a romantic comedy being filmed in Paris, but you're having trouble with the love scenes because you're falling in love with the film's delicious director. After several takes, it's obvious that you're a bit distracted.

The Climax: As you make your way to the bed on set once more, the director tells everyone to call it a wrap. Distraught and confused, you ask, "But why? We have all day to get this right." Taking your hand, the director replies, "I know, but I'm going crazy watching you kiss another person. Today, I hope you'll let me have you all to myself."

The Phantasm: Monk and Follower

The Setting: You are a monk who has been asked to provide spiritual counseling to a follower who's struggling with the faith. You're prepared to guide the follower through the process of unlocking the mind and body from worldly desires when you find yourself gazing into the follower's gorgeous, soul-searching eyes. Despite years of asceticism, you can barely contain yourself.

The Climax: Your loins stirring, your talk is cut short when you hear the follower say, "I want to be pure, but I'm having trouble abstaining with all the wicked thoughts filling my head. I wish there was some way I could be satisfied without being really naughty." You're pretty sure that there's a way to be saucy without being sinful, as you slowly start to insert Burmese bells (a.k.a., Ben wa balls), slippery with lube, into this horny, lost soul's pulsating hole, one by one, and, at the moment of climax, you pull on the cord.

Going "Kink"

Hedonism just gets hotter when it comes to misbehaving. BDSM, which breaks down into bondage/discipline (B&D) and sadomasochism (S&M), is erotic power play that develops from the tension between domination and submission. While people tend to think that the individual being dominated is helpless, the power roles are actually equal. The submissive person has as much power as the dominant, if not more in that this partner calls the shots on how far things go and when it's game over. Freeing for both partners, the center of these exchanges is power and desire. Some people, in fact, never actually have sex, focusing instead on eroticizing each other in other ways. Seduction and mutual pleasure are the main game, and BDSM:

➜ Cranks up your sex life for years to come, fighting boredom and fostering monogamy.
➜ Helps you become better communicators.
➜ Keeps things creative.

➜ Invites greater intimacy through more personal exposure.
➜ Can make you feel more wanted and taken care of in your relationship.
➜ Enables you to test your physical and emotional limits in a safe space.
➜ Teaches you about yourself—and your partner.
➜ Releases you physically and emotionally for sweet sexual surrender.
➜ Deepens trust that strengthens bonds between lovers.

You may be thinking that your lover would never go for something this out of the mainstream when it comes to sex play, but he or she might surprise you. This is what Drew discovered: "My girlfriend was shy the first time she brought up her submissive fantasies. We had just finished having sex, and she said that she likes to think of herself as my 'slave.' It was hard for her to say that, but it turned me on, too, and since then, we have incorporated that role-play into our sex life. I love it."

As with all of the topics we've covered in this book, you need to make sure that your relationship can handle this kind of daring adventure. When talking about erotic power play, you should discuss any vulnerability and trust issues that can make it hard to let go and fully enjoy the experience. Part of doing this may involve discussing power dynamics that are already playing out in the relationship; for instance, one partner's controlling nature may tend to dominate what lovers do, where they do it, and when. Use the following questions to steer your conversation:

Are you both, individually, ready for erotic power play? A person must feel secure with him- or herself and feel healed from any past issues that could make him or her vulnerable in these exchanges. In figuring out if erotic power play is for you, ask yourself:

→ Am I sexually self-confident?
→ Do I see myself as desirable?
→ Do I like myself?

→ Will I accept myself in the dominant or submissive role?
→ Do I feel secure in what I would be doing?
→ Am I good at owning my own power and taking command? (Am I known as a good leader?)
→ When it comes to this kind of sex play, have I explored my needs for what I want to get out of the experience?

Should we go with B&D or S&M?
People tend to think that B&D and S&M are one and the same, but there are some slight differences. B&D focuses on symbolic or physical restraint, whether that's binding a partner's arms and legs with a restraint, such as handcuffs, or tying their appendages to an object, such as a bedpost. A body part may be constricted, as well. The partner in charge controls the submissive's behaviors at times, using discipline when necessary, based on rules and forms of physical or psychological punishment that partners have agreed upon in advance.

With S&M, the sadist is sexually gratified by inflicting mental or physical pain on a love object. The masochist is pleasured by the pain, humiliation, or domination inflicted by the love object. The sensations from S&M tend to be more intense than those in B&D, going beyond bondage to biting, scratching, pinching, whipping, etc.

Who should take what role? Discuss each other's interest in being the one in charge (the active, leading dominant "top") and the obedient one (the submissive "bottom"). In choosing your role, remember that these are not your primary identities outside of these exchanges—they are merely for your private playtime. Also, don't feel locked into what you select: People may have top or bottom preferences, but it's good to switch things up, especially in the first few experimental sessions.

To determine whether you'd make a good top, ask yourself:

→ Can I direct the behavior, suspense, and mystery and build anticipation by confidently teasing and tormenting?

→ Am I good at giving commands (e.g., "Get down!")?
→ Can I deliver sensations that might cause my partner pain?
→ Will I respect guidance from the bottom?
→ Do I realize that I'm not seeking mental or emotional control over my partner?
→ Do I like being nurturing and acting as a caretaker?
→ Do I enjoy the sensations that come with having power and control?
→ Can I responsibly handle the power and new feelings that will come about from being in control?

If you've determined you would make a good top, think about your answers to the following questions:

→ Will I punish "bad" behavior?
→ Will I use pain as punishment and how?
→ How will I build sensory anticipation?
→ How will I reward good service (e.g., give compliments for good behavior)?

→ Will I demand something nonsexual (e.g., a massage)?

→ Will I agree to switch roles at some point?

→ How will I provide sensation as the bottom assumes different positions (e.g., gentle strokes during spanking that gradually get more forceful as more blood fills the bum, fondling the genitals in between other forms of stimulation)?

To determine whether you'd make a good bottom, ask yourself:

→ Am I willing to set the session's basic conditions and the instructions that the top will follow?

→ Do I like relinquishing control to another?

→ Can I handle being told what to wear, how to pose, and how to service my partner?

→ Would it be fun and arousing to pretend to misbehave?

→ Can I respond to the action in a way that keeps things rolling and exciting?

→ Am I comfortable expressing how I feel?

→ Can I use the safe word we choose to halt all action when necessary?

What are your limits? As you define and negotiate your roles, it's important to set limits. The boundaries you establish must be understood and respected by your partner. Bring up your fears and concerns and talk about what aspects of erotic power cross the line for you.

What sorts of behaviors are okay? For example, consider these:

→ Pinching
→ Biting
→ Scratching
→ Tickling
→ Bondage
→ Spanking
→ Caning
→ Flogging
→ Hot temperatures (e.g., paraffin candle wax)
→ Cold temperatures (e.g., ice, stainless steel medical instruments)
→ Sucking sensations (e.g., vacuum cups)

Clarify what sensations feel good on which body parts and at what level of intensity.

Also, is verbal punishment, such as humiliation, okay? If it gets the green light, you need to put the sex talk skills you've acquired to good use. Discuss what types of verbal abuse are a turn-on (e.g., "I want you doing the nasty like the whore you are") and which will feel abusive (e.g., having your appearance or figure belittled). These preferences are very individual and come down to a number of factors, including emotional abuse one may have experienced in other relationships. So make sure you've hammered out what is and isn't allowed.

After discussing the physical and emotional pros and cons of all these elements, write up how you will treat and view one another during power play sex. Consider it a contract for psychological safety, knowing, however, that like your role, your preferences aren't set in stone. You can always change your mind about things like the intensity or level of pain desired.

A few last words of advice:

➜ When restraining your partner, make sure that the restraints are secure without being too tight.
➜ When your partner is restrained, check that he or she doesn't feel any stress on his or her muscles or joints.
➜ Never tie anything around someone's neck.
➜ Never leave arms or legs suspended for too long because it can cause numbing and discomfort.
➜ Never leave your partner alone.
➜ Have surgical scissors on hand in case of emergency and a tether needs to be cut.

Who are you playing and what's your storyline? Before you begin, decide whether you're going to be yourselves or take on characters. If you're taking a fictional route, pick out-of-the-ordinary names, such as Zara or Brooklyn. What accessories or costumes would add to the action (e.g., corset, spandex, stockings, rubber suit)? Dressing up can be quite a turn-on, as Mel can tell you: "An ex-boyfriend who I was still hooking up with was very turned on one day when I came over wearing high-heeled black boots. He ordered me to strip down to boots and panties only and then told me he was going to spank me. . . . But he did it *very* slowly and made me lie on his lap for a little bit first, then kept rubbing my ass and telling me I was going to get spanked, before finally doing it."

Slipping into a character role can be empowering in a way that's helpful when being risqué. Read through these storylines for inspiration:

→ Mistreated captive: It may seem cruel, but this captive needs to be taught a lesson in respect after a recent escape attempt. With your captive tied to down, you proceed to drip hot wax from a paraffin candle, making the skin tingle with discomfort, and ask if the foolish one is going to pull such a stupid stunt again.

→ Rebellious niece: You wish that your live-in's niece had gone to Cancun for spring break instead of coming to visit the two of you. She's been rude, thankless, disrespectful, and has started to bring home guys and girls she's met at local bars. She needs to bend over and get what she deserves, followed by a good spanking. In fact, you can already hear the exchange: "Why am I punishing you?" Because I'm a bad girl. "And where do bad girls get punished?" In their . . .

→ Teacher in charge of detention: You were caught leaving school grounds and are now being forced to stay for detention. Only your punishment isn't writing "I will stay on campus" a thousand times on the chalkboard. The teacher in charge would much rather tie one of your arms to the desk and have you masturbate with your other hand, all the while tickling you with a light feather. You're not allowed to push it away, and if you try, you've been promised a good rap on the knuckles.

→ Intern for a powerful politician: You've moved to your country's capitol to further your dream of becoming a world leader one day.

While getting the staff coffee wasn't exactly you had in mind, you suddenly have access to a high-powered politician who appears to be checking you out. This is confirmed one morning when you accidentally spill iced coffee all over the politician's lap, only to hear: "No worries! Just help me get out of these wet clothes. Special favors often lead to more than getting me coffee, if you know what I mean."

What instruments of pleasure will you use? Whether you use something from around the house or purchase erotic power play gear, keep things safe. In addition to regular sex toys, you may want to play around with these items:

→ Wooden spoons
→ Clothespins
→ Ropes
→ Slappers
→ Handcuffs
→ Soft cuffs
→ Mattress restraints
→ Blindfolds
→ Gags
→ Soft floggers
→ Scarves
→ Neckties
→ Medical tape
→ Chains
→ Plastic wrap
→ Elastic bandages
→ Rulers
→ Wooden hairbrush
→ Metal spoons
→ Straps
→ Belts
→ Switches
→ Crops
→ Paddles
→ Bamboo rods
→ Spatulas
→ Canes
→ Paraffin candles
→ Vacuum cups
→ Medical instruments
→ Soft doe skin whips

Don't be surprised if you or your partner cries tears of grief or joy. These experiences are intense, and participants need to let it all out.

When coming down from your experience or responding to an emotional reaction, be supportive and affectionate.

Cuddle. Then, once things have calmed down, talk about what the experience was like for you: Would you be up for doing it again? What would you do differently?

Chapter 6 Check-In

As you process this chapter's material on fantasy and role-playing, consider these questions:

→ What potential do fantasy and role-playing have for giving your sex life new excitement and passion?
→ What did you like?
→ What didn't work?
→ What would you be eager to try again?
→ How would you do things differently?
→ Which scenarios held particular appeal for you? How would you tweak them to make them even hotter?
→ How did it feel to play certain characters?
→ Where you successful in communicating with your partner?

Finally, evaluate your erotic talk attempts. What was it like to talk about your fantasies and potential role-plays? What were you able to do that you may not have accomplished before you read this book? Where did you succeed in weaving in some smoking sexy talk? What are you most definitely planning on doing again?

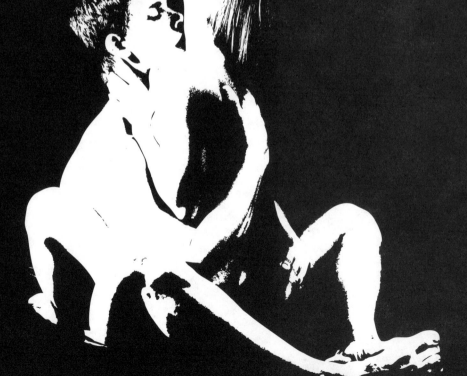

"Give me
more."

Tackling Issues That Can Trump Your Game:
Shedding Sexual Inhibitions and Issues

IN CHAPTER 7, YOU'LL LEARN HOW TO:

✔ Size up major factors that may be inhibiting you from letting loose, aurally speaking.

✔ Break through barriers impacting erotic talk.

✔ Assess your sexy talk success so far.

"I'm a great public speaker, an effective communicator, and confident when it comes to expressing myself . . . except when it comes to erotic talk. It's like the cat's got my tongue. Every word feels like a weight, and it's more effort than erotic for me. I'm sure it has to do with my upbringing around sex. We hardly said the word, let alone talked about such matters."

DOES THIS SENTIMENT from Devon feel familiar? Whether you regard yourself as a total rookie or quite advanced in the auditory department, a huge factor in how you've reacted to the exercises in this book boils down to your ability to give yourself permission to be sensual. It also comes down to our ability to let go of the rules of carnal conduct that govern our sensuousness. Whether we realize it or not, we're affected by all sorts of agents when it comes to exuding our sexual nature (or not)—some of which date back to our earliest years.

From society to those who raised us, any number of traditional influences can discourage us from seeking our pleasures, let alone outright owning them in our vocal reactions. So in this chapter, you and your lover are going to undo the bondage of the unsexy kind that's been sabotaging your sex life, taking on the potential barriers to becoming babelicious during your erotic talk attempts. We're going to tackle the major personal issues and communication challenges that can get in the way of talking sexy and sex talks.

You in the Lingo Limelight

I've been teaching university human sexuality classes for well over a decade. And whether I'm working with an eighteen-year-old undergrad or a fifty-five-year-old graduate student, I've found that my class is often the first opportunity people have to explore how they've come to be the sexual person they are today. For a variety of reasons, few individuals have been given the opportunity, or dared to roll up their sleeves, to think about influences that have shaped their sexuality and relationships.

In making this most exciting, personal expedition, you'll look at your innermost sexual makeup as well as the dynamics that govern the limits of your relationship with your lover. The process requires a mix of brutal honesty, heart, and courage, plus a willingness to identify and overcome obstacles. The holy grail you get in the end is priceless: By undoing the gag suffocating your sound, you'll free yourself to take risks and tap your sexual core for a more satisfying relationship.

Personal Inhibitors that Become Passion Killers

You likely know them well—those personal inhibitors that trump our ability to talk about sex or have sexy talk. They read like a rap sheet: body image issues, feelings of anxiety, shame, guilt about sex and sexual expression, and problems experiencing touch and affection. The damage done is enormous. Anyone suppressing their sexuality and desires may worry that they'll seem naïve when talking sexy. They may feel vulnerable, scared, or uncomfortable at the prospect of emotionally exposing themselves. Others may worry about being dismissed, misunderstood, or unheard. All of this goes for those with a great deal of sexual experience and very little alike.

Trip knows how difficult and nerve-racking it is for some to talk about their sexual wants, needs, fears, and issues: "We don't engage in sexy talk very often, honestly—not as often as I would like, and certainly not as often as we should. My lover suffers from depression, body, self-confidence, and in turn, libido issues. All of this causes problems in our relationship, though she refuses to acknowledge it. I try to explain to her that my desire for erotic talk is about reclaiming our lost intimacy and not about the lost sexual satisfaction or release. I feel the need to be intimate and wish she'd at least be willing to talk about how we can be truly sexually intimate again."

Personal inhibitions can quickly extinguish erotic talk efforts, putting out any hope in our ability to make sex better. If sex talks are awkward, difficult, ultimately unsatisfying, and anything but sexy, they all too easily make better sex a backburner effort instead of a priority.

But if you're determined to benefit from everything this book has to offer you and your relationship, both of you need to tackle what's at play, despite feeling intimidated or uncomfortable. You need to learn how to express your "stuck" emotions and unmet or unacknowledged needs positively if you expect to coax your sexual nature as never before. This starts with not allowing yourselves to feel guilty or shameful for wanting sensual and sexual pleasure; it's something we all have a right to pursue and enjoy.

For this exercise, we're going to deal with the energy drainers blocking you when it comes to expressing yourself sexually. Journaling can be a very effective way to sort through your thoughts, get your feelings out there, and shed light on how to move forward. You may want to run through this list in a single sitting, or you may prefer to focus on one item at a time, returning to the others when you feel recharged and ready to examine underlying issues at play. Consider this personal reflection one of the best sex gifts you can ever give to yourself. Address these topics in your journaling:

1. What are your earliest memories of the opposite sex, same sex, nudity, and genitals?

2. What are your earliest memories about the sexual atmosphere in your home (e.g., nudity, sleeping habits, bathing, masturbation)?

3. How did you learn about vaginal-penile intercourse? Anal intercourse? Oral sex? What did you think of each initially? Over time?

4. What was puberty like for you (e.g., first ejaculation or first menstrual period, growing up with social pressure, body changes)?

5. Write about your first love. (Note: Anything goes, even a pet or teacher.)

TIME: 30 minutes

LUST-INDUCING LOCATION: anywhere you can be alone with your thoughts (e.g., on a blanket in a park or in your private study space)

MATERIALS: journal and pen

PEAKING POTENTIAL: 0.5—some reflections can awaken your libidinal energy

6. How do your feelings about your body play into your ability to be verbally and nonverbally expressive with a lover?
7. Do you express or contain your sexual energy as it builds? Why do you react in such a way?
8. How would you describe your sexual self, or the sexual/erotic side of your personality?
9. What would you identify as energy drains when it comes to realizing your full sexual potential? Consider your gender, sexual orientation, religious teachings, parental messaging, peer influences, etc.
10. What sorts of behaviors, sensations, emotions, circumstances, etc., would make for some of the best sex of your life? (In other words, what are the whos, whats, whens, wheres, and whys of different scenarios that turn you on?)

Feel insightful? Hopefully, your answers hold wisdom about what controls your sex life—understandings that you can use to change patterns, unlock emotions and desires, and derive more pleasure and excitement from your relationship.

Whether you keep your journal private or share your responses with a lover is up to you. Some people find it cathartic to burn these journal pages and fire up new passions, while others discover the upside of letting their partner in on their intimate thoughts, like Casey did: "My initial erotic talk effort was in the form of a journal entry written while my boyfriend was away on vacation without me. Although there were lots of very intimate thoughts not relating to sex, after he read the journal, the only thing that got mentioned was the sex talk bit and an exploration from him as to whether I would engage in my fantasy threesome. At least it was a start."

How You Might Be Hurting Your Own Game

Let's be honest: Everyone has their good sides and less than desirable sides. When it comes to the quality of the sex communication in your relationship, you may be concerned, annoyed, or frustrated if your partner is less than enthusiastic about erotic talk, but consider—and I say this not knowing you—that you may also be part of the difficulty. You are one-half of a relationship and therefore must take responsibility for your role. You must do what's necessary to make your partner want to come out and aurally play.

To find out just how supportive and accessible you are (or aren't), finish the following sentence: "My partner would probably characterize my communication style as . . ."

→ Nagging
→ Bossy
→ Whiny
→ Sugary
→ Impatient
→ Dominating
→ Blaming

Whether you selected one or all of these adjectives to finish the sentence, it's an indication of a problem in the relationship. All these communication styles stir up negative energy, which only invites adverse reactions.

If your partner sees you as someone who is always complaining, bickering, etc., he or she won't feel comfortable opening up, let alone go anywhere near erotic talk. Fearing your blame, rejection, or criticism, they'll retreat, and the relationship (not to mention the sex) will suffer as negative feelings fester and resentment builds. Sound familiar? For your sake, I hope not, but awareness is the first step toward creating change and having the type of sexual sharing that you want.

Now that you're aware of your own shortcomings, ask yourself: What can I do to improve the situation for a sexually charged atmosphere? What do I need to change about the way I interact with my partner to get to a better place that enables us to strip down about intimate issues, like sex— a place where erotic talk feels fun and natural?

Becoming more self-aware, understanding what your tendencies are and the impact they have on your partner, is a major step toward realizing your erotic talk goals. It's about evaluating the kind of energy you bring to your relationships, for better or for worse. As you confront your communication style and make yourself more receptive to changing what doesn't work, barriers will come down. Trust will deepen.

Erotic talk efforts will become easier as you become increasingly fearless, clear, encouraging, and open with each other. This translates into a sexier you—the supremely sexy you who inspires your lover's sexual energy.

The following exercise was inspired by Roger, who found that a mirroring approach to erotic talk was quite effective in supporting his lover: "To teach my wife how to express herself, I used a series of 'repeat after me' phrases. After a while, as we had sex, she was able to say what I wanted to hear without my taking the lead." This exercise also doubles as a way of learning how to be a good listener.

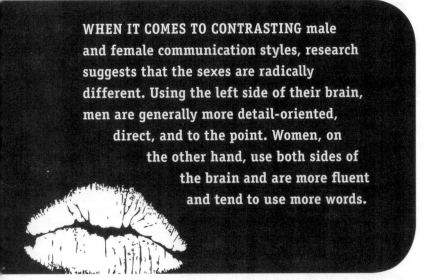

WHEN IT COMES TO CONTRASTING male and female communication styles, research suggests that the sexes are radically different. Using the left side of their brain, men are generally more detail-oriented, direct, and to the point. Women, on the other hand, use both sides of the brain and are more fluent and tend to use more words.

Make a list of all of the things you'd like to say to your partner and the things you would like to hear uttered from your lover's lips during a heated moment. For now, stick with statements that are affectionate, romantic, spiritual, or sensual. (Over time, you can move on to the seductive and hardcore if you wish—unless, of course, you're ready to charge ahead now. If so, go for it!) These statements may be compliments, requests, commands, ideas, etc.

Pick the phrases on the list you find easier to say, and ask your partner to repeat them after you. Allow yourselves to react truthfully, whether with stunned silence or laughter. Some expressions will not be easy to repeat, especially if they feel out of context. So allow these to come naturally—maybe during a breathless makeout session. Who can resist repeating things like the following when you're all wrapped up in one another and wanting more?

➜ "I love your body!"
➜ "I want you."

➜ "I want to feel you."
➜ "You make me so hot."
➜ "You're beautiful."
➜ "Let's get naked."
➜ "Your scent drives me crazy."
➜ "I only ever want to be inside you."
➜ "I could melt into you."
➜ "You're all I ever want."
➜ "You're so naughty. I love it."

TIME: 15–20 minutes

LUST-INDUCING LOCATION: anywhere you can privately exchange sensual sentiments, such as your bedroom

MATERIALS: pencil and paper

PEAKING POTENTIAL: 2—higher if it puts you in a frisky mood

Guys and Dolls: How Gender Limits Lip Service

I don't like to play up gender differences because, for the most part, males and females are much more alike than they are different. This is true in the bedroom as well. We share many of the same erotic needs and concerns, including those about safety, connection, trust, fantasy, challenge, passion, intensity, comfort, thrills, fears, etc.

IF YOU OR YOUR PARTNER is being held back by personal inhibitors or can't seem to engage each other through healthy communication, consider meeting with a sex therapist or counselor to work through the issues. For a sex therapist or counselor in your area, visit the American Association of Sex Educators, Counselors, and Therapists website at www.aasect.org.

But thanks to the "Mars-Venus" media rage that has been playing up "he said, she said" differences for years, we've been brainwashed to think that the sexes are worlds apart. The claim has been made, mostly by people with no formal training in sexuality or communication, that men are much better at certain forms of erotic talk than women. Sex writer Tracey Cox once wrote that "most men beat women hands down when it comes to talking dirty." On that, I would beg to differ. And the misconceptions we're about to hit on back me up.

MISCONCEPTION #1: MEN ARE SUPPOSED TO BE IN CONTROL OF THEIR EMOTIONS

Many guys are afraid to lose control in the sack. Thanks to social conditioning, they've gotten the message loud and clear that they're supposed to keep it together at all times, even as lovers. They've been taught that making noise means losing control, so men work to remain silent, even killing their sexual response in the process. The reluctance to attempt erotic talk stems, too, from the worry that he'll come across as too animalistic, much to the chagrin of lovers like Chris: "To hear a strong and sexy man plead for me to fuck him is a major turn on—to know he wants me more than anything at that time drives me insane. When it comes to the silent type, it's like doing the dead."

Many men see sex itself as a voiceless way to express emotions. This is especially true for men who have trouble articulating their feelings or making themselves vulnerable. This reluctance to open up is reinforced by the societal notion that talking about sex isn't a "guy thing," as Lana knows: "I talk about sex all the time, but then again I'm a female. . . . My boyfriend would rather eat a gun than talk about his, my, or our sexuality. So I turn to my friends when he's unresponsive."

MISCONCEPTION #2: A MAN SHOULD KNOW WHAT TO DO IF HE LOVES ME.

How many times have we heard this one before? "If he loved me, he'd know what to do." Too many hetero-sexual couples have been plagued by the Prince Charming scenario, with the Snow Whites of the world waiting, hoping, and praying for all of their erotic needs to be met. Those in same-sex relationships are no better off when it comes to this myth. We've been taught that our dream lover always performs to perfection. And in this, women have been brainwashed to think that we're little more than sexual responders to his superior efforts.

PUH-leeze. The idea that women are supposed to be delicate damsels, void of desire until a man shows up to stoke the flames of passion irritates me to no end. Not only is the quality of sex compromised because it takes two to tango, but it also takes two to reach new levels. The best sex happens when lovers are actively engaged in fulfilling their own as well as their partner's desires. Being in tune with and attending to your wants, needs, and yearnings is what leads to satisfaction—and knowing what you want and what pleases you is incredibly sexy.

MISCONCEPTION #3: GREAT MALE LOVERS DON'T NEED FEEDBACK

Related to the previous misperception is the idea that true studs can ride their lover like they drive their car. They don't need directions. They always know what they're doing—with anyone. *Not!* Anybody who thinks that a person knows how to be a great lover without instruction or feedback needs to think again. Sex doesn't work that way. We're all different, and what made one lover swoon won't necessarily have the same effect on the next. And men can come away baffled and confused when a new partner is unresponsive to a technique that wowed their last lover.

When you talk to their partners—and I have—the other side of the story emerges, and the unfortunate consequence of buying into this myth is laid bare. Things aren't working; the technique, the style, the approach . . . it isn't quite right. Yet their partners are afraid of insulting or hurting their lover by expressing this.

The simple truth is that we don't come with an instruction manual. So if you find yourself guilty of this fallacy—and not having the quality sex that you'd like—it's time to become your own personal sex tour guide, offering your lover a one-of-a-kind, once-in-a-lifetime safari of your hottest destinations. If you don't, you deprive yourself of the opportunity to explore and express your sexuality as you make your way to becoming sexually fulfilled.

MISCONCEPTION #4: ONLY SISSIES COMMUNICATE THEIR FEELINGS AND NEEDS

A major assumption about male sexuality is that it's feminine and weak to talk about feelings and needs, as women are known to do. The cruel irony is that research has found that the highest levels of marital satisfaction are associated with the presence of shared "linking" traits that are regarded as more "feminine" in both genders.

These include being nurturing, caring, affectionate, sympathetic, gentle, kind, and devoting oneself to others. Research has further confirmed that both sexes prefer a feminine approach to providing comfort, seeing this as more effective in supplying emotional support.

Married or not, don't let yourself be duped by the sissy stereotype. Sexy lovers are those who express themselves often and honestly. You will only reap rewards by letting your guard down and sharing your soft side; think of it as engaging in a little "sexposure."

MISCONCEPTION #5: GOOD GIRLS DON'T LIKE IT DIRTY

If she's virginal, innocent, classy, sweet, or angelic, then the belief is that she shouldn't be listening to dirty talk like "Eat me 'til I squirt all over your face." She's too pure for it. This myth is bad for good sex because women who consider themselves "good girls" have trouble getting down and dirty.

Adding to the problem, their lovers fear that it's an insult to utter impurities or beg these women for them, like

Bradley: "As a heterosexual guy, it's very hard for me to talk dirty. I came of age around a lot of gender-equality and feminism, which I value and believe in entirely. It took me a long time to accept that I can value a woman as an equal, while simultaneously thinking of her as a sex object. It is still difficult for me sometimes, even in my thirties. Therefore, although I want it and I love it, usually my girlfriend has to begin the dirty talk for me to feel comfortable with it. She understands this and she does it."

MISCONCEPTION #6: ONLY "CHEAP" WOMEN ENGAGE IN EROTIC TALK

Women seen as demanding, overly aggressive, or unladylike when it comes to sex get pegged with some harsh labels, as are women who are sexually assertive, go after what they want, and communicate their needs. This happens in spite of the fact that being vocally sexpressive is more acceptable for women than for men. Tradition holds that good girls are supposed to keep their legs crossed and their traps shut when it comes to having sex.

As a consequence, some women grow into adulthood unwilling to ask for what they want in bed or to express their sexual exhilaration for fear of being seen as cheap. The impact of being verbally and sexually inhibited can extend to their lovers, who pay the price for their reluctance to get into erotic talk. Listen to Jon, "I love all kinds of erotic talk. The more the merrier. I just wish more women were comfortable doing it. And, not just doing it, but doing it because they *want* to do it and not because they are acting out something they think their man wants. There's nothing worse than a person half-heartedly talking dirty!"

Sexually active women need more encouragement and guidance in expressing their sexual needs, desires, and preferences—and often, women need to be taught how to be in charge of their sexuality. (This goes for men who are timid when it comes to erotic talk as well.) All lovers stand to gain a great deal by sharing their intimate sex-on-the-brain details and what's going to make for hotter, more amazing sex. Getting it out there with respect to what works leads to greater comfort with each other and better results, as couples find themselves happier and more sexually responsive than ever.

Sexual Orientation: Who Has It Easier?

When it comes to sex communication, word on the street has been that nonheterosexuals are seasoned pros—with lesbians better than therest. This conventional wisdom is supported by research showing that sexually active gays and lesbians have more open, effective communication than heterosexuals. Detailed findings include:

→ Nonheterosexuals are likelier to talk more easily, openly, and often about the kinds of sexual activities they do and don't enjoy.
→ Gays and lesbians use more affection and humor in addressing a disagreement, with their partners more positive in how they receive it. They're also better at staying positive after a disagreement than straight couples.

- The positive comments of gay and lesbian partners have more of a "feel good" impact than they do for heterosexual lovers.
- Lesbian relationships exhibit more humor, anger, excitement, and interest than gay relationships when partners fight.

These findings are helpful in shedding light on how gay or lesbian couples communicate, but they don't necessarily mean that homosexuals are better at erotic talk or excused from sex talks simply because they're dealing with familiar territory. In other words, it's dangerous and misguided to assume that if you're gay or bisexual, you know what your partner likes because you're used to operating with the same equipment.

Consider instead that studies have found that relationship satisfaction is the same across all sexual orientations, indicating that same-sex couples do not actually have this perceived advantage. We're all individuals when it comes to our sexual wants, desires, and needs, regardless of gender or sexual orienta-tion. Lovers, gay or straight, need to be proactive in talking to their partners about their sexual preferences and dislikes if they're interested in a lifetime of superior sex.

Family Ties that Can Stifle Sexual Expression

Anyone reared in a home where sex was barely mentioned or discussed in negative terms lacks a positive model for talking about anything sexy. For those who were raised to view sex as dirty or immoral, sex communication of any kind can be embarrassing and unthinkable, and something to avoid. Even a family's ability to communicate in general can have an impact on your comfort level in expressing yourself. Cherise explains: "I hate to bring my family into it, but I was raised in a house where the only feelings that were expressed were usually those that had been bottled up for so long. We just never expressed our wants or desires or dreams, outside of 'I'd like chicken tonight.' "

You or your partner may be dealing with the issue that sex is a zip-your-lips topic, as was the case for Shawn: "My ex and I were rather reserved verbally with each other around sex in large part because of his Catholic upbringing and his lack of confidence. I would moan and make sounds. He was silent. Only rarely would one of us use the 'F word' during lovemaking. After we went our separate ways, I became very sexually active and experimented with letting everything go. I make more noise now. I say anything and everything depending on my partner and the mood. It makes a world of difference."

It takes time to undo the damage created at home. In some cases, it may require individual or couples' counseling or therapy, and in others, couples will simply need to be patient as lovers unlearn lessons from childhood. Moreover, those raised in communicative families may realize that they need to take the lead in the couple's sexy talk efforts, as was the case for Nick: "I was raised in a very verbal family. My wife was not. It took her a while to become comfortable expressing herself verbally. She is sexually introverted, so it is difficult for her to express herself—her

wants and desires. My talking to her helps her see how freeing it can be. It helps her explore her own vocalizing, which is all very exciting to me."

When you assume this type of leadership role, you will find it gratifying when partners respond to your efforts. Reactions like Macey's can be motivators: "Since my upbringing was so inhibited, I branched out when I got involved a partner who was more open with his sex communication. Also, confidence and knowing myself as I get older helps!"

The ethnic group you belong to can have an impact on your ability to talk about sex. Research has found that Asian American couples are less likely to discuss sex, as are Hispanic American couples. Further, Hispanic and African American people rely more on nonverbal communication, especially touching, than European Americans in revealing sexual information.

Exercise: Overcoming Obstacles to Lusty, Lasting Intimacy

You and your lover should complete each of the following sentences individually and then compare answers. As you discuss your responses, frame your answers along the lines of how influences, like family, have impacted your communication abilities for better or for worse.

1. When I think about self-disclosure or revealing myself to another, I . . .
2. When conflict occurs with another, I . . .
3. One way I show affection is by . . .
4. I have trouble expressing myself when . . .
5. Miscommunication has gotten me into trouble in . . .
6. My greatest strength as a communicator is my ability to . . .
7. The biggest challenge I've faced in communicating with people I've been attracted to has been . . .

While processing everything we covered in this chapter, think over the last six chapters and the exercises you've attempted. Which ones would you like to revisit? What strengths do you have in making sure that your efforts and those of your partner are launched this time? What issues do you need to keep in check to own your sexuality and your ability to express yourself?

Now that you have a better understanding of issues that might be hampering your efforts, get empowered. Take a stand and refuse to let them interfere with or infringe upon your pleasuring. Sexual rights are human rights, and you have every right to express yourself erotically!

TIME: 15 minutes

LUST-INDUCING LOCATION: your bed

MATERIALS: pad of paper and pen

PEAKING POTENTIAL: 0—although opening up to each other often stirs feelings of tenderness and connection

Chapter 7 Check-In

This chapter was tough, so congrats on sticking it out! In evaluating how you did in this chapter, answer the following:

1. What, if anything, is influencing your ability to engage your lover in different forms of erotic talk? Will any of this require more work given the established boundaries? Will any issues require professional help for you or your partner (e.g., the prospect of being unable to avoid communication is scary for some)?

2. Do you feel better about the possibilities for self-disclosure in your relationship?

3. If your efforts are still proving difficult, personally or for your partner, what strengths and tools can you harness and expand? What work needs to be done to boost your efforts?

4. How successful do you feel about your erotic talk efforts? How far have you come since page 1?

CONCLUSION

The End Is Just the Beginning

Something tells me that now that you know the upside of erotic talk, you'll never want to keep your mouth shut when getting sexy again. By taking in everything this book has to offer, you are well on your way to becoming accomplished in the art of aural sex. After all, you've:

➜ Embraced the role of sound in sex, seduction, and eroticizing your relationship.
➜ Discovered how sound and certain words and phrases can awaken your mind and amplify your sexual response.
➜ Learned to express yourself erotically, from panting to putting it out there.

You know a lot more about erotic talk than the average lover, and your partner is surely impressed with how adept you've become. I know I am. Aural efforts aren't easy, but the payoffs are huge! With your verbal charm galore, you've become a better, hotter sex communicator who is now more confidently, comfortably in charge of your pleasuring. Among a whole host of other skills of the sexually adept, you now know how to increase sexual desire, share your sexual fantasies, and flirt like a champ.

You now have the ability to launch your sex life with even more tongue action. You have the power to up your satisfaction and eroticism. What you've mastered in these pages will enable you to milk the benefits of erotic talk, such as keeping your relationship fresh, fun, faithful, full of surprises, and always sexy. Language has the power to enchant, and the spells you've learned to cast are sure to amplify your pleasure, intensify your feelings, and enhance your sexual experiences, as well as those of your lover.

But your efforts don't end here. This book is just a naughty and necessary pit stop in your journey to greater passion and more meaningful relationships. So in steering your efforts from here, ask yourself: What were the main highlights? How was I successful? What am I looking forward to doing again or doing differently? What ideas do I have that we didn't touch on?

From here on out, you'll have your partner hanging on your every word.

RESOURCES

Books of Erotica

Alison Tyler's erotica collection

Anne Rice's erotica collection

The Black Lace Book of Women's Sexual Fantasies, edited by Kerri Sharp (Virgin Black Lace, 2003)

Erotic Fantasies for Romantic Couples, by Bella Beaudoin (PublishAmerica, 2003)

Erotica: Women's Writings from Sappho to Margaret Atwood, edited by Margaret Reynolds (Ballantine Books, 1998)

Harlequin novels

Je T'Aime: The Language of Love for Lovers of Language, by Erin McKean (Portico, 2008)

Ladies' Home Erotica, by the Kensington Ladies Erotica Society (Ten Speed Press, 1984)

The Mammoth Book of Best New Erotica, by Maxim Jakubowski (Running Press, 2007)

Nancy Friday's erotica collection

Online Lit and Writing Resources

Clean Sheets: An Online Erotic Magazine, www.cleansheets.com

Erotica Readers & Writers Association, www. erotica-readers.com/ERA/index.htm

Literotica.com (free sex stories, erotic audio, adult fiction)

Other Books by Yvonne K. Fulbright, Ph.D.

The Better Sex Guide to Extraordinary Lovemaking, by The Sinclair Institute (Quiver, 2010)

The Hot Guide to Safer Sex, by Yvonne K. Fulbright (Hunter House, 2003)

Pleasuring: The Secrets to Sexual Satisfaction, by Dr. Yvonne K. Fulbright (Hollan Publishing, 2008)

Sex with Your Ex & 69 Other Things You Should Never Do Again . . . Plus a Few That You Should, by Dr. Yvonne K. Fulbright (Polka Dot Press/Adams Media, 2007)

Touch Me There! A Hands-On Guide to Your Orgasmic Hot Spots, by Dr. Yvonne K. Fulbright (Hunter House, 2007)

Your Orgasmic Pregnancy: Little Sex Secrets Every Hot Mama Should Know, by Danielle Cavallucci and Dr. Yvonne K. Fulbright (Hunter House, 2008)

Sex and Sexuality Information

Go Ask Alice!
www.goaskalice.columbia.edu
Columbia University's health Education Program; Q&A site

San Francisco Sex Information
P.O. Box 881254
San Francisco, CA 94188-1254
www.sfsi.org
415.989.7374 or 877.472.SFSI (7374)
Provides frequently asked questions, weekly columns, and referrals

Sensualfusion.com
Offers sex Q&A, sex coaching and education services

Sexuality Information & Education Council of the United States
www.siecus.org
212.819.0109
Nonprofit organization providing sex education programs and materials

Sexuality Source
www.sexualitysource.com
(or www.yvonnekfulbright.com)

Offers sex education, writing, and consulting services and a free newsletter

Online Erotica Retailers

Adam and Eve, www.adameve.com

Condomania, www.condomania.com

Eve's Garden, www.evesgarden.com

Good Vibrations, www.goodvibes.com

Sexuality Source Enhancements Store, www.sexualitysource.com

Sinclair Institute, www.sinclair.com

Toys in Babeland, www.babeland.com

Sexual Health

The Hot Guide to Safer Sex , by Yvonne K. Fulbright (Hunter House, 2003)

Sexual Health Network
3 Mayflower Lane
Shelton, CT 06484
www.sexualhealth.com

World Association for Sexual Health,
www.worldsexology.org

The Women's Sexual Health Foundation,
www.twshf.org

Sexual Pleasuring

*The Clitoral Truth: The Secret World
at Your Fingertips*, by Rebecca Chalker
(Seven Stories Press, 2000)

The Complete Manual of Sexual Positions,
by Jessica Stewart
(Sexual Enrichment Series, 2003)

How to Have Good Sex
www.howtohavegoodsex.com

*Pleasuring: The Secrets to Sexual
Satisfaction*, by Dr. Yvonne K. Fulbright
(Sterling, 2008)

*The Sinclair Institute's Better Sex Guide
to Extraordinary Lovemaking*,
by Dr. Yvonne K. Fulbright (Quiver, 2009)

*Taboo: Forbidden Fantasies for Couples,
by Violet Blue (Cleis Press, 2004)*

*Touch Me There! A Hands-On Guide
to Your Orgasmic Hot Spots*,
by Dr. Yvonne K. Fulbright
(Hunter House, 2007)

Tantric Sex

The Art of Sexual Ecstasy, by Margo Anand
(Putnam, 1989)

The Art of Tantric Sex, by Nitya Lacroix
(DK, 1997)

Tantric Love, by Ma Ananda Sarita and
Swami Anand Geho (Fireside, 2001)

Tantric Sex for Women, by Christa Schulte
(Hunter House, 2005)

ACKNOWLEDGMENTS

While this is my seventh book, doing acknowledgments never gets old. My warmest thanks to the team at Quiver Books for their hard work and feedback—William Kiester, Jill Alexander, and Nancy King. We've made healthy communication one red-hot read!

A special thank-you also goes to everyone who helped me to officially launch my business, pursue a postdoctoral fellowship, and write two books in the past year . .

➜ My wonderful family, who inspire me in all that you do: Charles G. Fulbright, Ósk Lárusdóttir Fulbright, Anna Huld Lárusdóttir, Sveinbjörn Hafliðason, Sigurður Snævarr, Eydís K. Sveinbjarnardóttir, Þórunn Sveinbjarnardóttir, Anna Sveinbjarnardóttir, Silla Thorarensen, and Sveinbjörn Thorarensen.

➜ Dr. Sóley Bender, for taking me under your wing and giving me the opportunities of a lifetime.
➜ Frances Harber, for escapes to the Blue Lagoon and for welcoming me into your home.
➜ Sean Duffy and Ásgeir Sigfússon, for good times over glasses of wine.
➜ All of my friends and colleagues, for always rallying behind my efforts and spreading the word.

Many thanks, too, to everyone who boldly filled out the Erotic Talk Survey. Your personal thoughts and anecdotes were so appreciated.

And last, but certainly not least, enormous thanks to Dave Saquet for his encouragement, energy, love, and support. It all means more than you know.

ABOUT THE AUTHOR

Yvonne K. Fulbright, Ph.D., M.S.Ed.

Originally from Iceland, sexologist, sex educator, and relationship expert Dr. Yvonne K. Fulbright is the author of several books about sex and relationships. A popular media resource, she has been featured in hundreds of media outlets around the globe, and is the sex columnist and sex expert for *Cosmopolitan* magazine and Foxnews.com. Yvonne is also a monthly contributor to disaboom.com and professor of human sexuality at Argosy University. In 2004, she founded of Sexuality Source, Inc., a communications and consulting organization specializing in the topics of sex, sexual health, sensuality, and relationships. For more information on Yvonne, her projects, and sensual fusion coaching services, visit www.sexualitysource.com.